OCCUPATIONAL HEALTH NURSES AND RESPIRATORY PROTECTION

IMPROVING EDUCATION AND TRAINING

LETTER REPORT

Committee on the Respiratory Protection Curriculum for
Occupational Health Nursing Programs

Board on Health Sciences Policy

Linda Hawes Clever, M. E. Bonnie Rogers,
Andrea M. Schultz, and Catharyn T. Liverman, *Editors*

INSTITUTE OF MEDICINE
OF THE NATIONAL ACADEMIES

THE NATIONAL ACADEMIES PRESS
Washington, D.C.
www.nap.edu

THE NATIONAL ACADEMIES PRESS • 500 Fifth Street, N.W. • Washington, DC 20001

NOTICE: The project that is the subject of this report was approved by the Governing Board of the National Research Council, whose members are drawn from the councils of the National Academy of Sciences, the National Academy of Engineering, and the Institute of Medicine. The members of the committee responsible for the report were chosen for their special competences and with regard for appropriate balance.

This study was requested by the National Institute for Occupational Safety and Health of the Centers for Disease Control and Prevention and supported by Award No. 200-2011-38580, T.O. #1, between the National Academy of Sciences and the Centers for Disease Control and Prevention. Any opinions, findings, conclusions, or recommendations expressed in this publication are those of the author(s) and do not necessarily reflect the view of the organizations or agencies that provided support for this project.

International Standard Book Number-13: 978-0-309-21548-0
International Standard Book Number-10: 0-309-21548-X

Additional copies of this report are available from The National Academies Press, 500 Fifth Street, N.W., Lockbox 285, Washington, DC 20055; (800) 624-6242 or (202) 334-3313 (in the Washington metropolitan area); Internet, http://www.nap.edu.

For more information about the Institute of Medicine, visit the IOM home page at: **www.iom.edu.**

The serpent has been a symbol of long life, healing, and knowledge among almost all cultures and religions since the beginning of recorded history. The serpent adopted as a logotype by the Institute of Medicine is a relief carving from ancient Greece, now held by the Staatliche Museen in Berlin.

Suggested citation: IOM (Institute of Medicine). 2011. *Occupational health nurses and respiratory protection: Improving education and training: Letter report.* Washington, DC: The National Academies Press.

*"Knowing is not enough; we must apply.
Willing is not enough; we must do."*
—Goethe

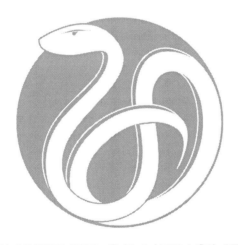

INSTITUTE OF MEDICINE
OF THE NATIONAL ACADEMIES

Advising the Nation. Improving Health.

THE NATIONAL ACADEMIES
Advisers to the Nation on Science, Engineering, and Medicine

The **National Academy of Sciences** is a private, nonprofit, self-perpetuating society of distinguished scholars engaged in scientific and engineering research, dedicated to the furtherance of science and technology and to their use for the general welfare. Upon the authority of the charter granted to it by the Congress in 1863, the Academy has a mandate that requires it to advise the federal government on scientific and technical matters. Dr. Ralph J. Cicerone is president of the National Academy of Sciences.

The **National Academy of Engineering** was established in 1964, under the charter of the National Academy of Sciences, as a parallel organization of outstanding engineers. It is autonomous in its administration and in the selection of its members, sharing with the National Academy of Sciences the responsibility for advising the federal government. The National Academy of Engineering also sponsors engineering programs aimed at meeting national needs, encourages education and research, and recognizes the superior achievements of engineers. Dr. Charles M. Vest is president of the National Academy of Engineering.

The **Institute of Medicine** was established in 1970 by the National Academy of Sciences to secure the services of eminent members of appropriate professions in the examination of policy matters pertaining to the health of the public. The Institute acts under the responsibility given to the National Academy of Sciences by its congressional charter to be an adviser to the federal government and, upon its own initiative, to identify issues of medical care, research, and education. Dr. Harvey V. Fineberg is president of the Institute of Medicine.

The **National Research Council** was organized by the National Academy of Sciences in 1916 to associate the broad community of science and technology with the Academy's purposes of furthering knowledge and advising the federal government. Functioning in accordance with general policies determined by the Academy, the Council has become the principal operating agency of both the National Academy of Sciences and the National Academy of Engineering in providing services to the government, the public, and the scientific and engineering communities. The Council is administered jointly by both Academies and the Institute of Medicine. Dr. Ralph J. Cicerone and Dr. Charles M. Vest are chair and vice chair, respectively, of the National Research Council.

www.national-academies.org

COMMITTEE ON THE RESPIRATORY PROTECTION CURRICULUM FOR OCCUPATIONAL HEALTH NURSING PROGRAMS

LINDA HAWES CLEVER (*Co-Chair*), California Pacific Medical Center, University of California, San Francisco

M. E. BONNIE ROGERS (*Co-Chair*), Occupational Safety and Health Education and Research Center, University of North Carolina at Chapel Hill

EDIE ALFANO-SOBSEY, Wake County Human Services, Raleigh, North Carolina

BARBARA DEBAUN, Cynosure Healthcare Consultants, San Francisco, California

OISAENG HONG, Occupational and Environmental Health Nursing Program, University of California, San Francisco

LESLIE M. ISRAEL, Department of Medicine, University of California, Irvine

JAMES S. JOHNSON, JSJ and Associates, Pleasanton, California

HERNANDO R. PEREZ, Drexel University School of Public Health, Philadelphia, Pennsylvania

PATRICIA QUINLAN, School of Medicine, University of California, San Francisco

Study Staff

CATHARYN T. LIVERMAN, Study Co-Director
ANDREA M. SCHULTZ, Study Co-Director
LARISA M. STRAWBRIDGE, Research Associate
JUDITH L. ESTEP, Program Associate
ANDREW M. POPE, Director, Board on Health Sciences Policy

Reviewers

This report has been reviewed in draft form by individuals chosen for their diverse perspectives and technical expertise, in accordance with procedures approved by the National Research Council's Report Review Committee. The purpose of this independent review is to provide candid and critical comments that will assist the institution in making its published report as sound as possible and to ensure that the report meets institutional standards for objectivity, evidence, and responsiveness to the study charge. The review comments and draft manuscript remain confidential to protect the integrity of the deliberative process. We wish to thank the following individuals for their review of this report:

Felicia Bayer, Alcoa, Inc.
Lisa M. Brosseau, University of Minnesota School of Public Health
Kathleen Buckheit, North Carolina Occupational Safety and Health Education and Research Center, University of North Carolina at Chapel Hill
Howard J. Cohen, Independent Consultant
Karen Coyne, U.S. Department of the Army
Sue L. Davis, College of Nursing and Health, University of Cincinnati
Joanna Gaitens, University of Maryland School of Medicine
Elaine L. Larson, Columbia University School of Nursing

Although the reviewers listed above have provided many constructive comments and suggestions, they were not asked to endorse the conclusions or recommendations, nor did they see the final draft of the report before its release. The review of this report was overseen by **Ada Sue Hinshaw,** Graduate School of Nursing, Uniformed Services

University of the Health Sciences. Appointed by the Institute of Medicine, she was responsible for making certain that an independent examination of this report was carried out in accordance with institutional procedures and that all review comments were carefully considered. Responsibility for the final content of this report rests entirely with the authoring committee and the institution.

Contents

Acronyms

AAOHN	American Association of Occupational Health Nurses
ABOHN	American Board for Occupational Health Nurses
ADN	associate degree in nursing
AIHA	American Industrial Hygiene Association
ANA	American Nurses Association
ANSI	American National Standards Institute
APIC	Association for Professionals in Infection Control and Epidemiology
BSN	baccalaureate of science in nursing
CDC	Centers for Disease Control and Prevention
CFR	Code of Federal Regulations
CM	case management
COHN	certified occupational health nurse
COHN–S	certified occupational health nurse–specialist
ERC	Education and Research Center for Occupational Safety and Health (NIOSH)
HRSA	Health Resources and Services Administration

ICOH	International Commission on Occupational Health
IH	industrial hygiene
IOM	Institute of Medicine
LLNL	Lawrence Livermore National Laboratory
NFPA	National Fire Protection Association
NIOSH	National Institute for Occupational Safety and Health
NPPTL	National Personal Protective Technology Laboratory
NSSRN	National Sample Survey of Registered Nurses
OHN	occupational health nurse
OSHA	Occupational Safety and Health Administration
PHRST	Public Health Regional Surveillance Team
PPE	personal protective equipment
RN	registered nurse
SM	safety management
UCLA	University of California, Los Angeles
UCSF	University of California, San Francisco

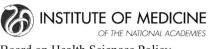

INSTITUTE OF MEDICINE
OF THE NATIONAL ACADEMIES

Board on Health Sciences Policy

August 2, 2011

Maryann D'Alessandro
Associate Director for Science
National Personal Protective Technology Laboratory
National Institute for Occupational Safety and Health
Centers for Disease Control and Prevention
626 Cochrans Mill Road
Pittsburgh, PA 15236

Dear Dr. D'Alessandro:

At the request of the National Personal Protective Technology Laboratory (NPPTL) of the National Institute for Occupational Safety and Health (NIOSH), the Institute of Medicine (IOM) appointed the ad hoc Committee on the Respiratory Protection Curriculum for Occupational Health Nursing Programs under the auspices of the IOM's Standing Committee on Personal Protective Equipment for Workplace Safety and Health. The overarching charge to the ad hoc committee was to examine existing respiratory protection curricula in occupational health nursing programs and to develop recommendations to improve education and training on the selection (including situation assessment), use, care, and maintenance of respirators. More specifically, the committee was asked to identify the essential content that should be included in occupational health nursing education and training programs and to recommend best approaches for teaching that content.

The committee's findings and recommendations for improving the respiratory protection curricula for occupational health nursing programs are summarized in this letter report. After gathering and reviewing the available information and evidence, including samples of existing respiratory protection curricula and content provided by NIOSH-supported Education and Research Centers for Occupational Safety and Health (ERCs), the committee concluded that occupational health nurses (OHNs) are

1

front-line advocates for preventing illness and injury and protecting and promoting health in the workplace. As key members of the occupational and environmental health and safety workforce, they contribute to the nation's health and productivity by mobilizing the knowledge, experience, and commitment of professional nursing to serve and help protect employees. OHNs work with employees in a wide array of settings that are associated with a diverse range of exposures and hazards, including agriculture, construction, health care, manufacturing, mining, services, trade, transportation, oil and gas extraction, and public safety. The role of OHNs is particularly important in protecting the respiratory health of America's workforce, and respiratory protection needs to be a consistent component of nursing programs at all levels.

Through its work, the committee determined two types of essential components of the occupational health nursing curriculum related to respiratory protection. One is technical and includes hazard assessment; selection, use, care, and maintenance of respirators; medical evaluation and monitoring; and fit testing. The second pertains to behavior: to best serve the health of nurses, workers, and the public, the technically oriented material must be paired with education on ways for nurses to protect themselves from respiratory exposures and hazards, the potential consequences of not using appropriate personal protective equipment (PPE), strategies for effective behavioral change and leadership, and strategies to build a culture of safety. The committee found that respiratory protection content taught in occupational health nursing programs receives varying amounts of dedicated time and resources and is taught using a variety of didactic and practical approaches. To improve the respiratory protection curricula for OHNs, the committee makes seven recommendations that are detailed in this report. Box 1 summarizes the committee's recommendations, which speak to the following areas: the responsibilities of OHNs, respiratory protection education and training, and incentives for respiratory protection education and training.

BOX 1
Recommendations

The Responsibilities of OHNs

Recommendation 1: <u>Conduct a Survey of OHNs</u>
The American Association of Occupational Health Nurses (AAOHN), working in collaboration with NPPTL and other agencies and professional organizations,

---

BOX 1 Continued

should conduct a survey of a representative group of OHNs asking about their current roles and responsibilities relevant to respiratory protection and asking for their input on education and training needs in this area.

Recommendation 2: Achieve and Maintain Knowledge and Skills in Respiratory Protection
OHNs should take responsibility for achieving and maintaining knowledge and skills in respiratory protection that are appropriate to their scope of practice. They should provide instruction and demonstrate leadership in motivating others to use respirators appropriately.

Respiratory Protection Education and Training

Recommendation 3: Expand Respiratory Protection Education Across All Levels of Nursing Education and Training
Nursing education programs across all levels, including licensed practical or vocational, diploma, associate, baccalaureate, and graduate levels, should

- introduce the basic concepts of respiratory risk and protection early in the education and training programs and throughout the curriculum;
- reinforce this knowledge when the students begin their clinical education and are fit tested for respirators;
- require that their graduates have a working knowledge of key elements of respiratory protection at the appropriate level for their scope of practice; and
- look to core curricula offered by occupational health nursing graduate and continuing education programs, including the NIOSH ERCs, for guidance on required knowledge and skills to educate nurses at appropriate levels for their scope of practice.

Recommendation 4: Ensure Essential Respiratory Protection Content in Occupational Health Nursing Graduate Curricula, and Adapt and Apply It to Continuing Education Programs and to the Education and Training of All Nurses
Occupational health nursing educators–in collaboration with staff from other disciplines (e.g., industrial hygiene, occupational medicine, engineering), NIOSH, AAOHN, and other expert sources–should ensure that essential respiratory protection content is included in graduate occupational health nursing programs and integrated into continuing education courses for OHNs. The essential respiratory protection content should

- reiterate the value of respiratory protection in reducing illness and injury;
- reinforce respiratory protection throughout the graduate occupational health curriculum and clinical practice;

Continued

BOX 1 Continued

- include content on hazard assessment; respirator selection, use, care, and maintenance; medical evaluation and monitoring; respirator fit testing; employee training; and program evaluation;
- require, at a minimum, familiarity with relevant federal (e.g., 29 CFR 1910.134), state (e.g., California Division of Occupational Safety and Health 5144), and national consensus (e.g., American National Standards Institute/American Industrial Hygiene Association Z88.10) regulations and standards;
- use hands-on education and training experiences to provide an understanding of the types of respirators and their uses;
- require students to demonstrate knowledge and skills in developing a respiratory protection program that includes training and evaluation components;
- emphasize the leadership role of OHNs in establishing a culture of safety, influencing behavior change and decisions related to respiratory and overall health, and promoting proper use of respirators in the workplace;
- examine research and best practices relevant to respiratory protection, behavioral change and leadership, and establishing a culture of safety in the workplace;
- consider including spirometry certification as a requirement for graduation; and
- specify elements that could be adapted and applied to continuing education programs and to the education and training of all nurses.

Recommendation 5: <u>Develop, Expand, and Evaluate Innovative Teaching Methods and Resources to Establish Best Practices</u>
Occupational health nursing education programs and respiratory protection programs should do the following:

- Integrate essential content on respiratory protection into their core curricula and continuing education programs through a variety of innovative approaches, taking into consideration the needs of the students. These methods could include

  o online courses (including webinars),
  o simulation techniques,
  o case studies,
  o education and training modules,
  o field observation and practice, and
  o conferences and workshops.

- Draw on resources available from NIOSH, the Occupational Safety and Health Administration, state and local governments, the NIOSH ERCs and other educational institutions, professional organizations and unions, advocacy organizations, international health and safety

BOX 1 Continued

organizations (e.g., the Network of World Health Organization Collaborating Centres in Occupational Health and the International Labour Organization), contractors, other professional communities and institutions, and the private sector.

- Collaborate with NPPTL to evaluate innovative teaching methods used for respiratory protection education and training, including continuing education, in order to establish best practices in the field.

Recommendation 6: <u>Expand Online Resources, Particularly Case Studies</u>
NPPTL should develop and maintain online resources for respiratory protection that are relevant to educating and training OHNs, specifically by

- developing template modules that could be used in the core curriculum for occupational health nursing programs and that would draw on best practices of the NIOSH ERCs (sections of these modules could also be used for nursing students at all levels);
- compiling case studies (e.g., health hazard evaluations) that illustrate the value of respirators in protecting the health of workers across a range of work environments; and
- providing easily accessible links to existing resources, including the OSHA checklists.

Incentives for Respiratory Protection Education and Training

Recommendation 7: <u>Explore the Development of a Set of Core Competencies in Respiratory Protection</u>
NPPTL, in collaboration with relevant professional organizations, should explore the development of a set of interdisciplinary core competencies in respiratory protection that could be used to guide the education and training of OHNs and other occupational health and safety professionals.

We would like to thank NPPTL and its staff members for generously supporting this study and for the guidance and information they provided to the IOM committee in the course of its work. We are also appreciative of the time and energy that the IOM committee and staff members dedicated to planning the successful information-gathering workshop that was held in March 2011 and to developing the report and its recommendations. We hope that NPPTL will find the committee's recommendations and this report informative as it considers ways to improve the respiratory protection curricula for OHNs and other occupational health and safety professionals.

Linda Hawes Clever, *Co-Chair*
M. E. Bonnie Rogers, *Co-Chair*
Committee on the Respiratory Protection Curriculum
for Occupational Health Nursing Programs

CHARGE TO THE COMMITTEE

Protecting the health of workers who are employed in workplaces with hazardous exposures (including chemicals, biologics, noise, radiation, particulates, stress, heat, and ergonomics) (NIOSH, 2011a) involves a range of protective measures that aim to remove the hazard or, if that is not possible, to mitigate the extent of the exposure through environmental-, administrative-, or individual-level measures. PPE standards and practices (including the use of hearing protection devices, respirators, gloves, eye protection, and protective clothing) are the primary means of hazard reduction and worker protection in some work situations and a key component for many others (e.g., chemical plants, mining, health care). With its mission to "prevent work-related injury, illness, and death, by advancing the state of knowledge and application of personal protective technologies" (NIOSH, 2009), NPPTL has explored the issues involved in respiratory protection through a number of IOM studies, which have supported the value of PPE use, including respirators, for the protection and promotion of worker health and safety (see Appendix C). Additionally, the IOM Standing Committee on Personal Protective Equipment for Workplace Safety and Health has had discussions on the range of professions, including occupational health nursing, that have an impact on improving the use of PPE.

NPPTL requested that the IOM conduct a study to examine respiratory curricula in occupational health nursing programs and make recommendations for essential content that should be incorporated into the curricula and approaches for teaching that content (see Box 2). This letter report and its findings and recommendations represent a starting point in a larger effort to improve respiratory education and training opportunities for all occupational health and safety professionals.

To respond to NPPTL's request, the IOM convened the nine-member ad hoc Committee on Respiratory Protection Curriculum for Occupational Health Nursing Programs. The committee included members with expertise in occupational health nursing and medicine, PPE design and training, industrial hygiene and occupational health, clinical medicine, and nursing education (see Appendix D for committee biographies).

BOX 2
Statement of Task

The IOM will conduct a study that examines respiratory protection curricula in occupational health nursing programs. The IOM committee will begin by examining the current respiratory protection curricula and training approaches used by the NIOSH ERCs and other occupational health programs. Based on this review, the committee will develop recommendations to improve training on the selection (including situation assessment), use, care, and maintenance of respirators. It will aim to address the following questions:

- What essential content should be incorporated in occupational health nursing education and training programs to produce professionals who are fully aware and informed about respiratory protection technologies?
- What are the best approaches for teaching that content so that effective respiratory protection programs are implemented?

As part of its data-gathering activities, the committee will plan and conduct a public workshop with input from the ERCs and relevant professional organizations, along with input from staff of health care and other employers where occupational health nurses are involved in training staff on respirator use. The committee will produce a letter report with its findings and recommendations.

STUDY PROCESS

The committee used several methods to reach its conclusions and recommendations. In addition to reviewing materials the committee held three meetings. The first meeting designed the study plan, began to gather and review available information, and started to plan a public workshop. The committee's second meeting included a public workshop held on March 30, 2011, in Pittsburgh, Pennsylvania, in conjunction with the NIOSH Personal Protective Technology Program's annual stakeholder meeting (see Appendix A for the IOM workshop agenda and Appendix B for a list of registered attendees). The workshop was an information-gathering session. Presentations from and discussions with experts provided the committee with insights about occupational health and safety, respiratory protection, and occupational health nursing. Workshop presenters discussed respiratory protection curricula currently used across the country, continuing education opportunities for OHNs, the role of professional boards or organizations in shaping occupational health nursing curricula, the on-the-ground perspectives of OHNs working in industry and health care settings, and challenges and opportunities for improving respiratory protection education and training for OHNs. At the third meeting the committee reviewed and edited the report draft and refined findings and recommendations.

To inform its deliberations and gain a better understanding of respiratory protection curricula, the committee received and reviewed the results of an NPPTL-led survey of respiratory protection curricula from six NIOSH ERC occupational health nursing programs[1] and from the North Carolina Division of Public Health.[2] The committee also reviewed the core curriculum and competencies of the American Association of Occupational Health Nurses (AAOHN). A literature search was conducted, but few articles currently exist on the educational needs of OHNs both in general and specific to respiratory protection or on effective teaching methods for respiratory protection content. The committee reviewed a selection of available literature on occupational health nursing and respiratory protection programs.

The committee's statement of task required that it focus on respiratory protection and, more specifically, on the essential content of respiratory protection curricula and the best approaches for teaching that content to OHNs. Therefore, this letter report does not address broader questions related to areas such as the capacity and efficacy of occupational health nursing programs or the education pipeline for OHNs, nor does it consider or evaluate the education of other occupational health and safety professionals in respiratory protection. The committee recognizes that OHNs are often educated and trained in interdisciplinary programs and courses that are sometimes taught by other occupational health and safety professionals, such as industrial hygienists. The committee also recognizes that successful respiratory protection programs in the workplace often involve the work of interdisciplinary teams of occupational health and safety professionals that include OHNs. Although this report is focused on OHNs, the committee believes that many of its findings and

---

[1]The six ERCs that submitted information for the survey were the University of Alabama at Birmingham School of Nursing; University of California, Los Angeles, School of Public Health; University of California, San Francisco; University of Iowa, College of Public Health; University of Michigan School of Nursing; and University of South Florida College of Public Health.

[2]The North Carolina Division of Public Health developed a respiratory protection training program that is used for training local health department staff throughout the state. The course materials used for this program were provided, along with the ERC materials, as part of the survey conducted by NPPTL.

recommendations could be applicable to the education and training of other professionals involved in respiratory protection programs.

BACKGROUND

Nationwide, there are approximately 5 million employees, across 1.3 million employment settings, who are required to wear respirators as part of their jobs (OSHA, 2011). A wide range of work environments may present respiratory health hazards to employees, such as the use of chemicals in agricultural and industrial settings, the presence of infectious agents in health care settings, and the presence of particulate matter in mining and construction settings. If effective safety and preventive measures are not in place, these exposures may negatively affect the health of employees and their families and could result in debilitating respiratory illness, disease, or death.

Collaboratively, industrial hygienists, safety engineers, OHNs, physicians, infection preventionists (called infection control officers in some workplaces), and other occupational health and safety professionals are responsible for monitoring workplace hazards; developing and implementing safety policies, procedures, and programs; educating employers and employees about occupational health and safety; complying with all relevant federal, state, and local regulations and standards; conducting workplace health assessments; and generally ensuring a safe working environment for all employees. Respiratory protection is one of many necessary components to ensure the overall health and safety of workers across employment settings.

Overview of Occupational Health Nursing

OHNs are nurses who work to prevent injury and illness and promote the health and safety of workers across a wide range of employment settings (IOM, 2000). Although OHNs make up a small proportion (< 1 percent) of the more than 3 million licensed registered nurses (RNs) in the United States (HRSA, 2010; Thompson, 2010), they represent the largest sector of health care professionals who work to ensure the health and safety of workers in employment settings (AAOHN, 2011).

In the course of their work, among many other tasks, OHNs act in the areas of management and organization, assessment, direct health care services to workers, prevention, and research. In management and organization, they may

- develop and implement occupational health and safety programs in the workplace;
- work to establish and maintain a culture of safety and health in the workplace;
- ensure compliance with federal, state, and other occupational health and safety regulations and standards; and
- contribute to emergency preparedness and disaster planning.

In assessment and direct health care services to workers, OHNs may

- assess and monitor the health status of employees relevant to their work responsibilities and work environments;
- help interpret medical diagnoses for employees and their employers;
- evaluate workers' medical and occupational history, health concerns, physical exams, laboratory results, and other health-related factors;
- document and treat occupational and non-occupational illnesses and injuries; and
- refer employees to employee assistance programs and other resources as needed.

In prevention and research, they may

- conduct assessments of employee health and workplace hazards;
- work to prevent occupational illness, injury, and death due to hazardous exposures;
- educate and counsel employees about occupational hazards and safety, healthy lifestyles and behaviors, and overall health and well-being; and
- conduct research to advance occupational health nursing and, more broadly, the field of occupational health and safety.

OHNs by the Numbers

The 2008 Health Resources and Services Administration (HRSA) National Sample Survey of Registered Nurses (NSSRN) estimated that there are 18,840 RNs whose principal nursing position is in an occupational health setting (HRSA, 2010). Since 1980, the number of OHNs in the United States has declined by approximately 36 percent, with 2008 representing the lowest number of OHNs in the last 3 decades (HRSA, 2010; Thompson, 2010). The 2004 NSSRN noted that, with an average age of 51 years, OHNs have the highest age among all of the settings in which RNs work (HRSA, 2006). In 2008, approximately 47 percent of OHNs were between the ages of 50 and 64 (HRSA, 2010).

Occupational Health Nursing Education and Training

OHNs come from a variety of educational backgrounds and have a wide range of professional experience. AAOHN, the profession's membership organization, conducts periodic surveys of its members. In a 2006 survey, AAOHN reported that approximately 42 percent of its members had between 6 and 15 years of occupational health nursing experience, 43 percent had greater than 15 years of experience, and only 15 percent had fewer than 6 years of experience (AAOHN, 2006a).

Generally, OHNs are RNs who provide occupational health nursing services; however, a small number of companies may hire licensed practical or vocational nurses to provide occupational health services. OHNs who are RNs can hold a diploma in nursing, an associate degree in nursing (ADN), or a baccalaureate of science in nursing (BSN)—the minimum levels of nursing education required to practice as an RN. Of those OHNs who are RNs, approximately 52 percent hold either a diploma or an ADN as their highest level of nursing education, whereas 30 percent have a BSN (HRSA, 2010). In 2006, AAOHN reported that approximately 11 percent of its members held a baccalaureate degree in another field (i.e., a non-nursing degree) as their highest level of education (AAOHN, 2006a).

Beyond basic nursing education, occupational health nursing specialty education is available at the master's and doctoral levels. Approximately 18 percent of OHNs have either a master's degree or a doctorate in nursing or a nursing-related field (not necessarily occupational health nursing) (HRSA, 2010). Graduate-level education may include programs of study as an occupational health nurse–specialist, an adult health nurse practitioner with a concentration in occupational health nursing, or a family health nurse practitioner with a concentration in occupational health nursing, such as the programs that are offered through the University of Michigan's Occupational Health Nursing Program (McCullagh,

2011). The largest contributors to graduate education and training in occupational health nursing are the NIOSH ERCs (IOM, 2000), which are typically part of an academic school of nursing or school of public health (see Box 3). In developing and implementing curricula for OHNs, graduate programs may use the core competencies and curriculum developed by AAOHN as a guide. The competencies are also used by the American Board for Occupational Health Nurses (ABOHN) to inform the development of the occupational health nursing certification exams. The AAOHN competencies are reviewed and updated every 4 years based on the evolving nature of the work environments, the practice of occupational health nursing, and the health care system (AAOHN, 2007). The overall course content in occupational health nursing programs, which was described in *Safe Work in the 21st Century* (IOM, 2000), generally corresponds with the current AAOHN core competencies (AAOHN, 2007) and curriculum (AAOHN, 2006b). The curricula and course content are reviewed and updated by the ERC occupational health nursing programs and submitted to NIOSH annually.

Continuing education also plays a large role in the education and training of OHNs. A wide array of continuing education courses in occupational health and safety exists for OHNs and other occupational health and safety professionals. Continuing education courses are offered through academic institutions, professional organizations such as AAOHN and the American Industrial Hygiene Association (AIHA), government agencies such as NIOSH and the Occupational Safety and Health Administration (OSHA), and private consultants. Continuing education requirements for maintaining nursing licensure vary by state. Further, professional organizations (e.g., ABOHN) that offer certifications set continuing education requirements for the specific occupational health nursing certifications that are available.

BOX 3
NIOSH ERCs for Occupational Safety and Health

NIOSH ERCs play a significant role in educating OHNs and occupational health and safety professionals. The ERCs were developed following the enactment of the Occupational Safety and Health Act of 1970 and the creation of NIOSH to, among other responsibilities, "help ensure an adequate supply of qualified professional occupational safety and health practitioners and researchers" (NIOSH, 2011c). To fulfill this mission, with NIOSH support

---

BOX 3 Continued

the ERCs conduct research and provide interdisciplinary graduate and continuing education opportunities across the continuum of occupational health and safety professions, including programs in occupational health nursing.

In the 2008-2009 academic year, there were 99 full-time and 64 part-time students enrolled in ERC occupational health nursing graduate programs (NIOSH, 2011c). Almost 82 percent of these nursing students were supported by NIOSH through stipends and tuition and fee reimbursement. Fifty-two OHNs graduated from ERC occupational health nursing programs in the 2009-2010 academic year. Nearly three-quarters of these graduates either secured employment in occupational health and safety positions or pursued additional graduate education in the field. Between 2005 and 2010, more than 200 OHNs graduated from ERC graduate degree programs (NIOSH, 2011c).

In addition to the occupational health nursing graduate programs, the ERCs also offer a number of continuing education courses for occupational health and safety professionals, including OHNs. These courses cover a broad range of topics across occupational health and safety and include courses in respiratory protection with topics such as fit testing. For example, in 2009-2010 one ERC, the Deep South Center for Occupational Health and Safety, offered 62 continuing education courses across the spectrum of occupational health and safety to over 1,300 participants (Oestenstad, 2010). During that same period, the University of Cincinnati ERC offered 322 courses with nearly 6,000 participants (Rice and Reponen, 2010). These courses were offered through traditional classroom settings and web-based learning.

Because of their dedicated focus on occupational health, these centers often offer respiratory education and training courses and/or incorporate them into their curricula. The ERCs may offer best practices in educating OHNs about respiratory protection. For this reason, ERC program directors and faculty along with their curricula played a large role in the information-gathering workshop and the committee's deliberations as the findings and recommendations for this report were developed.

Occupational Health Nursing Certifications

To demonstrate proficiency, OHNs have the opportunity to obtain certification credentials through ABOHN, which offers four certifications for OHNs—certified occupational health nurse (COHN), certified occupational health nurse–specialist (COHN–S), safety management (SM), and case management (CM). The COHN is designed for those OHNs who fill a clinical role, whereas the COHN–S has more of an emphasis on management and administration. See Table 1 for ABOHN certification requirements. According to the 2008 NSSRN, slightly less than

5,000, or approximately 26 percent, of OHNs report being certified in occupational health (HRSA, 2010).

TABLE 1 ABOHN Certification Requirements

Requirements	COHN	COHN–S	SM	CM
Active License	RN	RN	RN	RN
Education Minimum	diploma or associate degree	bachelor's degree	diploma or associate degree	diploma or associate degree
Active ABOHN Certification	N/A	N/A	COHN or COHN-S	COHN or COHN-S
Exam	150 multiple-choice questions	150 multiple-choice questions	200 multiple-choice questions	100 multiple-choice questions
Professional Occupational Health Experience	3,000 hours in occupational health in the previous 5 years or completion of an academic certificate of occupational health nursing	3,000 hours in occupational health in the previous 5 years or completion of an academic certificate of occupational health nursing or a graduate degree with a concentration in occupational health	• 25% of current position devoted to safety activities • 1,000 hours of safety experience in the previous 5 years	
Occupational Health Continuing Education	none	none	50 contact hours related to SM in the previous 5 years	10 contact hours related to CM in the previous 5 years

SOURCES: ABOHN, 2004, 2008a, 2008b, 2009.

RESPIRATORY PROTECTION ROLES
AND RESPONSIBILITIES

As described above, OHNs have a wide range of roles and responsibilities that span management and organization, worker health assessment and direct health care services, and prevention and research. Many, if not all, of these areas of responsibility may be applicable in some way to respiratory protection. Much like the overall roles and responsibilities of OHNs, the functions specific to respiratory protection vary widely and depend on the type of industry, the role OHNs play within the organization and within the occupational health and safety teams with whom they work, the level of resources and professional support available, the types of risks the workers face and characteristics of the workforce, and the OHNs' level of education and experience, among other variables.

The information presented at the workshop indicated great variability in the day-to-day responsibilities of OHNs. For example, OHNs may be involved in identifying, treating, and educating workers with possible respiratory diseases, monitoring worker health and lung function over time, developing respiratory protection policies for the workplace or employer, ensuring that individuals who have experienced a respiratory exposure with possible adverse health effects are appropriately treated and monitored, and encouraging the use of respirators when appropriate and in proper ways. The roles and responsibilities of OHNs across workplaces with active respiratory protection programs vary widely when it comes to fit testing, the selection and maintenance of respirators, and other aspects of respiratory protection. Some OHNs are involved in selecting and purchasing respirators, whereas others are not. Some conduct fit testing and select alternate respirators when a respirator fails a fit test for a worker. In other workplaces, OHNs do not perform fit testing at all because that responsibility belongs to another member of the occupational health and safety team. In some settings, OHNs are involved in respirator maintenance; elsewhere, this is the responsibility of an industrial hygienist.

Participants at the workshop highlighted additional roles and responsibilities relevant to respiratory protection that OHNs may assume, including

- providing leadership in promoting respiratory protection and bringing about behavior change in the workplace;

- being comfortable in educating and training fellow nurses and health care professionals about respiratory protection; and
- using worker respirator fit testing as a one-on-one opportunity to explain the importance of wearing a respirator and responding to other health risks and concerns as appropriate.

One core respiratory protection function that is often performed by OHNs is assessing workers' physical and psychological fitness to wear a respirator. OHNs therefore need to be familiar with conditions that frequently affect fitness, including hypertension, asthma, claustrophobia, and anxiety. Health assessments in the workplace also may provide opportunities to educate workers and promote health broadly, specifically for hypertension and other health risks. For example, during the workshop it was noted that cardiovascular limitations are a more common concern in medical clearances in workplaces than pulmonary function (Bayer, 2011). Although medical assessments offer the opportunity to address a range of health concerns, not all OHNs conduct these assessments. One reason is that states vary in their licensure regulations, which define scopes of practice for health care professionals and the types of health care services they may provide (IOM, 2011).

The function of OHNs within a workplace dictates not only their day-to-day responsibilities, but also the type of knowledge and skills that are required to effectively fulfill their duties. For example, OHNs who work in health care settings have specific knowledge needs that are different from those who work in a chemical plant or with workers in the agricultural industry.

Assessing the Respiratory Protection Roles and Responsibilities of OHNs

The primary methodologies used to understand the roles and responsibilities of OHNs are needs assessment surveys and practice analyses that are conducted by organizations such as AAOHN and ABOHN. These types of surveys are used to measure broadly the evolving nature of occupational health nursing work environments and the practice of occupational health nursing. The surveys are also used to inform the development and revision of competencies, to compare OHNs' actual tasks with the content of certification exams, and to ensure that OHNs and applicants for certification are being taught and tested on what they need to know to fulfill their roles and responsibilities.

In 2004, ABOHN conducted a practice analysis survey that drew responses from 794 certified and 429 non-certified OHNs (Strasser et al., 2006). The survey included 172 task statements, which were ranked on the basis of both significance and frequency. Although respiratory protection was not explicitly included as part of the survey, the top-ranking task statements that could have a respiratory protection component include "collaborate to protect and promote worker health and safety . . . apply regulatory standards and guidelines . . . conduct health surveillance for specific hazards . . . [and] monitor laws and regulations affecting nursing practice" (Strasser et al., 2006, pp. 19-20). Mackey and colleagues (2003) conducted an assessment of the educational needs of OHNs. The results provided information about the challenges and opportunities associated with graduate and continuing education of OHNs, and the assessment asked about the type of topics that would be of interest for their continuing education. However, respiratory protection was not explicitly included in the 25 topics identified on the survey, and spirometry[3]—one element of respiratory protection—was grouped with audiometry (Mackey et al., 2003).

Although there is a good understanding of the broad roles and responsibilities of OHNs as a result of the needs assessments and practice analyses conducted by AAOHN and ABOHN, these surveys include respiratory protection implicitly under larger rubrics, such as safety and injury prevention, regulatory compliance, and hazard surveillance. Therefore, not much is known about the day-to-day respiratory protection roles and responsibilities of OHNs.

A stronger understanding of the current respiratory protection roles and responsibilities of OHNs in their workplaces is needed to improve respiratory protection curricula and the teaching methods used in education and training. Therefore, a survey of OHNs that asks questions specific to respiratory protection would be beneficial to workers and occupational health nursing if it was conducted across a representative sample

---

[3]Spirometry is a test used to measure lung function. In the context of respiratory protection programs, spirometry is used for a variety of purposes that may include assessing workers' fitness for duty and assessing underlying pulmonary conditions (e.g., asthma) that may interfere with the proper use of a respirator. Spirometry is also used to establish a baseline of lung function, identify changes in lung function that may be a result of hazardous exposure in the workplace, and conduct surveillance and research on how specific hazards may affect lung function over time.

of OHNs who work in industries where respiratory protection is used. Questions that need to be asked include what proportions of OHNs are responsible for fit testing and spirometry, what proportions actively participate in respiratory hazard assessment, how many OHNs work in a setting where they are the only occupational health and safety professional, and how many work closely with an industrial hygienist, safety engineer, or other occupational health and safety professional on a regular basis. Additional questions could focus on education and training needs in respiratory protection and could include questions about challenges and barriers to achieving additional education and training, the preferred mechanism for receiving information on respiratory protection, and the preferred duration of respiratory protection courses that are offered. The results of this survey could be used to hone the content of respiratory curricula and to tailor teaching approaches to meet the needs of OHNs. The survey could be conducted online and could include a small number of focused questions. Additionally, it could be conducted as a public–private partnership between professional leadership and federal authorities.

Recommendation 1: <u>Conduct a Survey of OHNs</u>
AAOHN, working in collaboration with NPPTL and other agencies and professional organizations, should conduct a survey of a representative group of OHNs asking about their current roles and responsibilities relevant to respiratory protection and asking for their input on education and training needs in this area.

Responsibility to Ensure Safety

While job functions and responsibilities may vary from one OHN to another, there is one overarching responsibility that all OHNs, and all nurses, must fulfill: ensuring their own safety, the safety of their patients, and the safety of their families and communities. Provision 5 of the *Code of Ethics for Nurses* states:

> The nurse owes the same duties to self as to others, including the responsibility to preserve integrity and safety, to maintain competence, and to continue personal and professional growth. (ANA, 2010)

The responsibility to ensure safety for themselves, their patients, their families, and their communities requires that all nurses—from licensed practical or vocational nurses to advanced practice RNs, and including OHNs—know the value of respiratory protection and know when and how to properly use respiratory protection. This is of particular importance for nurses who work in health care settings and are frequently exposed to infectious respiratory hazards. These nurses have a responsibility to protect themselves against these hazards in order to stay healthy and to prevent the transmission of infectious respiratory diseases in their homes and communities.

In their day-to-day work and across their careers, ensuring safety is a vital responsibility of OHNs. Regardless of improvements that are made to respiratory protection curricula and teaching approaches for OHNs, overall advancements in respiratory protection cannot be made unless OHNs take responsibility for pursuing the necessary education and training. OHNs should have the knowledge and skills required to feel confident in using respiratory protection and teaching others to use it. Opportunities need to be available for respiratory protection and training, and individual OHNs need to use those opportunities to ensure that their knowledge and skills are up-to-date and appropriate for their scope of practice and the demands of their roles and responsibilities within their workplace.

> **Recommendation 2: <u>Achieve and Maintain Knowledge and Skills in Respiratory Protection</u>**
> **OHNs should take responsibility for achieving and maintaining knowledge and skills in respiratory protection that are appropriate to their scope of practice. They should provide instruction and demonstrate leadership in motivating others to use respirators appropriately.**

A Culture of Safety

By achieving knowledge and skills in respiratory protection, OHNs will be better equipped to fulfill their responsibility to ensure workplace safety. This responsibility also requires them to be educators, role models, and advocates for respiratory protection, working to establish and maintain a culture of safety—"an organization-wide dedication to the creation, implementation, evaluation, and maintenance of effective and current safety practices" (IOM, 2008, p. 120). When safety is a high priority, organizational-level environmental, engineering, and administrative controls join with individual-level behaviors to form a multidimensional program where the importance of worker safety is consistently reinforced (Hofmann et al., 1995).

Previous IOM reports have emphasized the importance of a culture of safety in establishing an effective worker safety program for health care workers. The 2008 report *Preparing for an Influenza Pandemic* highlighted "four key factors in promoting a culture of safety within healthcare facilities that are pertinent to PPE: (1) provide leadership, commitment, and role modeling for worker safety; (2) emphasize healthcare worker education and training; (3) improve feedback and enforcement of PPE policies and use; and (4) clarify worksite practices and policies" (IOM, 2008, p. 125). Occupational health professionals, including OHNs, have leadership and ethical responsibilities to work in collaboration with managers and other workers to create a culture of safety that promotes the value and proper use of respiratory protection. Academic preparation for effectively building and contributing to a culture of safety, with an emphasis on skills in leadership and collaboration, needs to begin in basic nursing education programs.

RESPIRATORY PROTECTION EDUCATION AND TRAINING

Improving the education of OHNs begins with ensuring that there is adequate respiratory protection content in basic levels of nursing education. The committee heard at the workshop that there is limited content on respiratory protection and, more broadly, on PPE and occupational health in basic nursing education curricula. As discussed above, all nurses have a responsibility to ensure safety. With regard to respiratory protection, this responsibility requires that all nurses know when and how to use respiratory protection properly. Therefore, nursing programs at all levels (licensed practical or vocational, diploma, associate, baccalaureate, and graduate) need to include instruction on respiratory protection at the level of specificity appropriate to the scope of practice. This instruction should include not only the "when" and "how" of wearing a respirator properly, but also an emphasis on the "why," which involves conveying the value of respiratory protection in health care work.

In basic nursing programs, content on respiratory protection could be included in employee and patient safety modules[4] and in disaster planning modules (Davis, 2011). When student nurses are being fit tested for respirators, these programs could also take the opportunity to explain when and why this equipment is important to their safety. Introducing respiratory protection content with an emphasis on its value early in basic nursing and clinical education could promote a better understanding of and respect for the importance of respiratory protection among all nurses, including those that go on to become OHNs. Additionally, having basic knowledge and skills in respiratory protection may promote a desire for additional education and training in that area.

Recommendation 3: <u>Expand Respiratory Protection Education Across All Levels of Nursing Education and Training</u>
Nursing education programs across all levels, including licensed practical or vocational, diploma, associate, baccalaureate, and graduate levels, should

- **introduce the basic concepts of respiratory risk and protection early in the education and training programs and throughout the curriculum;**
- **reinforce this knowledge when the students begin their clinical education and are fit tested for respirators;**
- **require that their graduates have a working knowledge of key elements of respiratory protection at the appropriate level for their scope of practice; and**
- **look to core curricula offered by occupational health nursing graduate and continuing education programs, including the NIOSH ERCs, for guidance on required knowledge and skills to educate nurses at appropriate levels for their scope of practice.**

Graduate-Level Curricula and Training

Across graduate-level education programs for OHNs, the content, duration, and level of specificity of courses that focus directly, and indirectly, on respiratory protection vary greatly. The committee's workshop

---

[4]Throughout this letter report, a module is defined as standalone, online content that is user friendly, is open source, and could be integrated into a curriculum.

provided an opportunity to hear from six ERC graduate programs on the components of their curricula that include topics related to respiratory protection. The committee also reviewed the information provided through an NPPTL survey of six ERCs and the North Carolina Division of Health. A summary of the information reviewed by the committee is provided in Box 4.[5,6]

In its review of the curricula, the committee identified the following common components of these programs relevant to respiratory protection:

- didactic courses on occupational diseases and injuries and on occupational hazard assessment that include information about respiratory illness and injury;
- a course on the fundamentals of industrial hygiene, which in some schools includes an overview of administering a respiratory protection program;
- respirator fit testing demonstrations and experience with information on assessing medical clearance for respirator use; and
- practicum experiences and/or field work, which in some cases includes respiratory protection.

Although the programs varied in the organization of the coursework and the requirements focused on respiratory protection, there was a common and notable interdisciplinary approach to education and training on respiratory protection. Interdisciplinary education is an intrinsic part of occupational health nursing graduate education because the practice of occupational health nursing is intertwined with the practice of industrial hygienists, physicians, safety professionals, infection preventionists, and others. Interdisciplinary coursework relevant to respiratory protection is often taught by industrial hygienists, including the respirator fit testing and spirometry sections of the course or module (see Box 4).

In reviewing the curricula, the committee found that spirometry courses, and in some cases in-depth respirator fit testing courses, are optional and usually involve additional expense to students. University of Alabama at Birmingham School of Nursing occupational health nursing students are encouraged and funded to take the continuing education program on respiratory protection programs and fit testing that provides

---

[5]The NPPTL survey results are available by request through the National Academies' Public Access Records Office.

[6]Slides from the workshop presentations are available online: http://www.iom.edu/nursesandrespirators.

didactic and participatory instruction (University of Alabama at Birmingham School of Nursing, 2011). Although spirometry is an optional course in some programs (e.g., Burns, 2011; Robbins, 2011); others, such as the University of North Carolina at Chapel Hill, require the spirometry course for graduation and course fees are covered (personal communication, M. E. B. Rogers, University of North Carolina, July 8, 2011). Both the cost of spirometry training and the time needed to teach it effectively were mentioned as barriers to offering a course as part of the required curricula. A survey of OHNs to better understand their roles and responsibilities, as described in Recommendation 1, could inform graduate programs as to whether spirometry should be a required part of the curricula.

Some of the programs that the committee heard about require graduate students to develop a complete respiratory protection program. At the University of California, Los Angeles (UCLA), for example, students are required to choose an industry and write a respiratory protection program relevant to that industry (UCLA School of Public Health, 2011). This requirement provides occupational health nursing students with the opportunity to better understand the various components of a respiratory protection program, strategies that can be used in planning and evaluation, and the challenges that may arise in developing and implementing an industry-specific program.

The committee also found that practicum requirements and hands-on experiences vary from program to program. Available practicum experiences may include an important opportunity for hands-on experience in respiratory protection. The 100-hour practicum in occupational health nursing required at the University of South Florida is precepted by a certified occupational health nurse practitioner or board-certified occupational medicine physician and includes worker teaching or counseling about PPE, which may include respiratory protection. Students are asked to consider whether the worker was wearing or using the PPE appropriately for the job when he or she was injured (Burns, 2011). As part of the occupational health nursing program at UCLA, graduate students participate in conducting respirator fit testing for undergraduate nursing students who are entering their clinical rotations (UCLA School of Public Health, 2011).

BOX 4
Overview of Respiratory Protection Curricula[a]

- **University of Alabama at Birmingham School of Nursing (Deep South Center for Occupational Health and Safety):** The fundamentals of industrial hygiene (IH) course, a 3-credit-hour course delivered as an online module, includes hazard assessment. There are also courses focused on occupational safety and ergonomics and adult health nurse practitioner content. Application courses include field interdisciplinary studies, worksite evaluations, practicum or residency, evaluation and management in occupational health, and spirometry certification. Students are encouraged to take the continuing education 3-day, in-person workshop, titled "Respiratory Protection Programs and Fit Testing," including hands-on and lecture content. Courses are taught by IH faculty.

- **University of California, Los Angeles, School of Public Health (Southern California ERC):** Respiratory protection content is threaded throughout the curriculum, with 8 hours dedicated to respiratory protection in the occupational health nursing theory course and additional time (of varying amounts) during clinical courses, practicums, or rotations. Students are given lectures on OSHA standards, hazard assessment, respirators, and worker protection programs. These courses are taught by occupational health nursing faculty with guest lectures by IH faculty. Students are required to write a worksite-specific respiratory protection program or the theory course final exam. Hands-on learning occurs when students participate in the fit testing of undergraduate nurses and during clinical rotations and plant visits. Students also take industrial hygiene and safety courses in the School of Public Health taught by IH faculty in which additional respiratory protection content is included.

- **University of California, San Francisco (Northern California ERC)[b]:** The course on health hazards in the workplace includes a demonstration of fit testing (2-3 hours). The program planning course includes the development of respiratory protection programs and staff training content (2 hours). In the course on occupational safety, respiratory protection content is covered (45 minutes). The clinical management of occupational health problems course includes content on spirometry interpretation (2 hours). An optional environmental health class includes a 1-hour section on respirators. Courses include presentations, informal content, and hands-on practice and are taught by IH faculty, safety professionals, and occupational and environmental health nursing faculty.

- **University of Cincinnati (University of Cincinnati ERC)[c]:** The occupational diseases and injuries course includes a 3-day NIOSH spirometry course and 3 hours on respiratory disorders (27 class hours). The course on management of occupational health programs includes designing a respiratory protection program using the OSHA standard (3 class hours). The

BOX 4 Continued

occupational exposure assessment course includes respiratory pro-tection programs, the OSHA standard, respirator types, medical clearance, and fit testing (3 class hours). Students have opportunities to do field work. Respiratory protection content is interdisciplinary, and IH faculty take the lead.

- **University of Iowa College of Public Health (Heartland Center for Occupational Health and Safety):** Respiratory protection content is first presented in the occupational and environmental health course with content including respirator basics, fit testing, equipment demonstration, and medical screening. In occupational health nursing courses, there are modules on PPE, respiratory questionnaires, and occupational spirometry. Students may take an optional spirometry certification course. The curriculum for the occupational health nursing practicum includes applying the modules of the courses listed above, including daily logs that track respirator activities, with 10-15 hours of instruction total (or more if the optional spirometry course is taken). Courses are taught by IH faculty.
- **University of Michigan School of Nursing (Michigan ERC):** The occupational and environmental health course includes respiratory disease and health effects content (2 credits, 16 hours). The introduction to occupational health course includes lectures and reading on hazard recognition and evaluation and exposure control, including respirator types, selection, fit testing, and training in use (3 credits, 15 hours, 2 hours of PPE content). Courses are taught by IH faculty.
- **University of South Florida College of Public Health (Sunshine ERC):** The occupational health nursing curriculum contains content related to respiratory protection equipment integrated throughout four required courses, including both lecture and field experiences. Twelve hours of lecture address properties, health effects, and control measures for aerosols, vapors, gases, and airborne particles. Fit testing, health promotion, and hazard and risk reduction are addressed. Classes, labs, and field experiences are taught by interdisciplinary faculty in IH, safety, occupational medicine, and occupational health nursing. Students can obtain certification in spirometry through completion of a 16-hour (lecture and lab) continuing education course conducted by occupational medicine faculty.
- **North Carolina Division of Public Health[d]:** This approximately 3-hour course includes didactic modules on respiratory hazards; respirator type, use; and donning and doffing; OSHA standards; fit testing; and PPE in health care settings. Students are provided with hands-on training for fit testing, respirator selection, and donning and doffing. Resources provided include a respiratory protection policy template, a medical evaluation questionnaire, and an evaluation checklist to enable health agencies to establish their own respiratory protection program. Courses are taught at the local health agency by IH instructors. Regional IHs are available to provide consultation and guidance on development and maintenance of their programs.

Continued

BOX 4 Continued

---

[a]Unless noted, detail was not provided on whether courses are required and the extent to which they focus on respiratory protection. Some programs included credit hours of a course, some included total hours spent in the course, and others included total time spent on respiratory protection (or PPE). Specific course names are listed where they were provided.
[b]The material was a written submission only; there was no workshop presentation by the University of California, San Francisco.
[c]The material was presented at the workshop only; there was no written submission from the University of Cincinnati.
[d]The material was a written submission only; there was no workshop presentation by the North Carolina Division of Public Health.

SOURCES: Brown, 2011; Burns, 2011; Davis, 2011; McCullagh, 2011; North Carolina Division of Public Health, 2011; Robbins, 2011; Rupe, 2011; UCLA School of Public Health, 2011; UCSF, 2011; University of Alabama at Birmingham School of Nursing, 2011; University of Iowa College of Public Health, 2011; University of Michigan School of Nursing, 2011; University of South Florida College of Public Health, 2011.

Continuing Education and Training

Many OHNs are likely to gain relevant knowledge and skills about respiratory protection through continuing education opportunities as the proportion who receive that information and training through their basic education and through graduate programs is currently limited. To educate the maximum number of OHNs about respiratory protection, targeted efforts need to be made to ensure the quality and efficacy of continuing education content and to promote the enrollment and completion of continuing education courses by OHNs.

Continuing education courses are typically short in length, ranging from a few hours to a few days, and are designed to improve and expand the knowledge, skills, and levels of expertise of OHNs. All NIOSH ERCs offer continuing education courses and programs for occupational health and safety professionals (NIOSH, 2011c). The ERC continuing education courses cover a wide range of topics and are offered through a variety of venues and use variable teaching approaches, such as professional conferences, traditional classroom settings, and online formats. Some courses are open to all occupational health and safety professionals, whereas others are specific to OHNs. Several examples of continuing education courses were presented at the committee's information-gathering workshop (Box 5).[7,8]

BOX 5
Overview of Continuing Education Courses
on Respiratory Protection

- **American Nurses Association (ANA):** The ANA provides training for first receivers of chemically contaminated victims and features some elements of respiratory protection. The ANA course is offered free of charge in both 1- and 3-day formats, and is taught by educators who travel to the students. The course includes content on respirator selection, uses, and limitations; OSHA best practices; medical clearance; fit testing; donning and doffing procedures; and maintenance and disposal of respirators. During the course, students have the opportunity to wear a powered air-purifying respirator (Carpenter, 2011).
- **M. C. Townsend Associates:** An independent consultant in the Pittsburgh area offers several courses, including a 1-day fit testing workshop, a 2.5-day NIOSH-approved spirometry course, and a 2-day spirometry refresher course and fit testing workshop (Townsend, 2011a). Much like those offered through the ERCs, these courses offer hands-on instruction and focus on the regulatory requirements relevant to respiratory protection (Townsend, 2011b).
- **University of Alabama at Birmingham School of Nursing:** The University of Alabama at Birmingham School of Nursing's Deep South Center for Occupational Health and Safety offers two continuing education courses that are specific to respiratory protection: a 2-day respiratory protection course, which was previously offered as a 4-day course, and a 4- to 6-hour fit testing workshop. In January 2011, the 2-day course included content on the following: a historical perspective on respirator use; respiratory hazards; respiratory protection program elements; standards, regulations, and guidelines; classification of respiratory protection equipment; breathing air quality and breathing air systems; respirator selection and use; respiratory protection program model outlines for public safety; medical evaluations; maintenance and care; record keeping; and programs and training for fit testing (University of Alabama at Birmingham School of Nursing, 2011). The fit testing workshop featured hands-on instruction and covered both quantitative and qualitative testing. Approximately one-quarter of the fit testing workshop participants were nurses, while only 1 percent of the participants who attended the 2-day

Continued

---

[7]The NPPTL survey of select ERCs did not explicitly cover continuing education content.
[8]Slides from the workshop presentations are available online: http://www.iom/nurses andrespirators.

BOX 5 Continued

respiratory protection course were nurses. Course surveys and follow-up questions from participants demonstrated that these courses are beneficial to the participants; however, feedback indicated that 2 days is not enough time to effectively cover the necessary content in the broader respiratory protection course (Maples, 2011).

- **University of North Carolina at Chapel Hill:** The North Carolina Occupational Safety and Health ERC at the University of North Carolina at Chapel Hill offers several continuing education courses that are designed for OHNs, two of which focus specifically on aspects of respiratory protection: "Respiratory Protection for Nurses" and "Pulmonary Function Testing" (a NIOSH-approved spirometry course). Other courses for OHNs, such as "Occupational Health Nursing. An Introduction and Review of Principles and Practice" and the OHN certification review courses, include some respiratory protection content, but the level of detail is variable. The "Respiratory Protection for Nurses" courseincludes the following components: anatomy and physiology; types of respirators; when and what types of respirators to use; how to use, store, and maintain respirators; qualitative and quantitative fit testing; medical clearance; and how to develop a respiratory protection program (Buckheit, 2011).

Challenges to Improving Respiratory Protection Education and Training

Across all levels of nursing education, the challenges in enhancing respiratory protection education and training include determining how to allocate time and faculty appropriately, identifying how to target the real-world needs of OHNs, and meeting the funding needs of the Programs in an affordable manner for students and employers. Challenges for students may include distance from programs and courses and a lack of understanding of the need or value of continuing education and training. For educators, insufficient interest or demand can present serious challenges to creating specialized courses with a narrow focus.

A major challenge faced by faculty in all nursing programs is how to allocate time in their courses and academic programs to ensure that all necessary content is covered (IOM, 2011). Additionally, decisions must be made about how to balance the importance of attaining a broad, general knowledge of occupational health and safety with including adequately detailed sections on more complex topics. Curricula at schools with occupational health nursing programs are already content rich and must cover a wide range of topics, including content on multiple types of PPE, such as hearing and eye protection, in addition to respiratory protection. At the graduate level, universities sometimes restrict the number of credit hours that a student can take per semester, which makes it difficult to add required courses without extending the time required to complete the program.

In addition to consideration of the type of content that should be taught and the level of detail that should be covered, decisions about who should teach the content can be complex. Clear distinctions cannot always be made between what content is directly within the purview of occupational health nursing in comparison to other disciplines, such as industrial hygiene and injury prevention. Interdisciplinary education offers advantages in laying the groundwork for collaborative practices (IOM, 2003), such as a close working relationship between a company's OHN (who might have primary responsibility for fit testing workers for respirators) and its industrial hygienist (who might have primary responsibility for hazard assessment and selecting and maintaining the respirators that are used). Although interdisciplinary education offers many potential benefits, implementing this approach can be challenging and requires additional time, coordination, and planning among faculty and administrators from the various professional programs. Further, it is challenging to fund specialized faculty for small numbers of occupational health nursing graduate students.

Another challenge is that education and training programs must appropriately tailor their courses to the needs of OHNs. OHNs work in a wide range of settings and have varying responsibilities. Therefore, graduate-level and continuing education programs must balance courses so that they impart both the knowledge and the practical skills needed by their graduates. As noted in Recommendation 1, obtaining further knowledge of OHNs' roles, responsibilities, and scope of practice in the workplace with regard to respiratory protection could provide opportunities to enhance education and training programs and help refine course content.

In addition, funding problems may exist for students and employers. Although financial support for some students is provided through the NIOSH ERCs or through employer tuition reimbursement programs, other OHNs and their employers may not have funding available to pay for graduate-level or continuing education courses. Mackey and colleagues (2003) found that more than a third of surveyed OHNs reported lack of money as an impediment to obtaining a graduate degree. Busy OHNs also may lack the time to participate in courses or may not be given time off by their employers for additional education. To attract participants, continuing education courses should be short in duration and affordable. Although availability of time and money are often key challenges, some OHNs and their employers may not see the need or understand the value of additional education in respiratory protection in the first place. Return-on-investment information and materials should be made available to nurses and their employers to clearly demonstrate the value of education and training in respiratory protection.

Essential Content of Respiratory Protection Education and Training for OHNs

Currently, respiratory protection content is taught in occupational health nursing graduate and continuing education programs using a variety of didactic and practicum approaches with varying amounts of dedicated time and resources. Additional information on the roles and responsibilities of OHNs, their educational and training needs, the perceived barriers to their achieving additional education and training, and their preferred educational approaches as they relate to respiratory protection will be valuable in efforts to improve the education and training of OHNs. The committee examined the existing programs and curricula, considered the applicable challenges to improving education and training, and participated in discussions throughout the workshop to identify the content that should be an essential part of respiratory protection education and training programs for OHNs. As a first step, the committee determined that a respiratory protection education and training program needs to

- be based on relevant federal, state, and other regulations and standards;
- include interactive and participatory components;
- emphasize the value of respiratory protection; and
- focus on leadership skills in promoting a culture of workplace safety.

Furthermore, OHNs need to be familiar with the OSHA respiratory protection regulations (29 Code of Federal Regulations [CFR] 1910.134) and how to implement them (see Ryan, 2001), as well as with other relevant federal and state (e.g., California Division of Occupational Safety and Health [Cal OSHA] 5144) regulations and national consensus stan-

dards (e.g., American National Standards Institute [ANSI]/American Industrial Hygiene Association [AIHA] Z88.10). The required components
that need to be in place for an employer's respiratory protection program
as noted in 29 CFR 1910.134 are

- "Procedures for selecting respirators for use in the workplace;
- Medical evaluations of employees required to use respirators;
- Fit testing procedures for tight-fitting respirators;
- Procedures for proper use of respirators in routine and reasona-
  bly foreseeable emergency situations;
- Procedures and schedules for cleaning, disinfecting, storing, inspect-
  ing, repairing, discarding, and otherwise maintaining respirators;
- Procedures to ensure adequate air quality, quantity, and flow of
  breathing air for atmosphere-supplying respirators;
- Training of employees in the respiratory hazards to which they
  are potentially exposed during routine and emergency situations;
- Training of employees in the proper use of respirators, including
  putting on and removing them, any limitations on their use, and
  their maintenance; and
- Procedures for regularly evaluating the effectiveness of the program." (29 CFR 1910.134)

In some workplaces, the OHN is the sole occupational safety and
health professional and serves as the respiratory protection program administrator. In this capacity, the OHN is required to implement all elements of a respiratory protection program—from hazard assessment to
respirator selection and maintenance—and would need to have a comprehensive knowledge of respiratory protection. In many cases, OHNs
are part of a team that implements the program and includes industrial
hygienists and safety professionals. Working in these circumstances requires a basic knowledge of respiratory protection.

Occupational health nursing programs need to be sure that students
have a basic understanding of and familiarity with all aspects of developing, implementing, and evaluating a respiratory protection program. Essential content of the occupational health nursing curriculum includes
education and training on hazard assessment; selection, use, care, and
maintenance of respirators; medical evaluation and monitoring; and fit
testing. Experience with both qualitative and quantitative methods of fit
testing is particularly useful. NIOSH could consider developing certified
respiratory protection courses for OHNs and other health and safety pro-

fessionals, similar to the NIOSH-approved spirometry course, which would incorporate observational assessments and demonstration of fit testing proficiency. A NIOSH-approved course of this nature could be offered in combination with the NIOSH-approved spirometry course.

Faculty in occupational health nursing programs should ensure that students are aware of specialty courses in respiratory protection that are available and should promote additional respiratory protection education and training through continuing education. Additionally, faculty should teach OHNs to recognize the limits of their education, training, experience, and scope of practice. For example, selecting a proper respirator and maintaining it in a workplace with a mixture of hazards is a complex undertaking that may require input from an industrial hygienist; selecting the wrong respirator can result in severe respiratory illness, disease, or death. Faculty should encourage and teach OHNs to work collaboratively with other experts in the field whenever possible and to seek out those experts when they are faced with circumstances that exceed their own knowledge and skill.

Technically oriented material in graduate programs should be paired with education on ways for nurses to protect themselves from respiratory exposures and hazards, consequences of not using proper PPE, strategies for effective behavioral change and leadership, and strategies to build a culture of safety and institutional support for respiratory protection. Understanding the value of respiratory protection is key to having a cadre of OHNs who can be leaders and champions in promoting the appropriate use of respirators in their workplaces. Courses on respiratory diseases and on identifying respiratory hazards can provide the necessary background and context. Essential content can be made more concrete through the use of relevant and timely case studies from workplaces, examples from U.S. and global environmental and occupational health issues, and journal articles that illustrate the value of and need for respiratory protection (e.g., Banga et al., 2011; CDC, 2010; Donham et al., 2011).

Recommendation 4: <u>Ensure Essential Respiratory Protection Content in Occupational Health Nursing Graduate Curricula, and Adapt and Apply It to Continuing Education Programs and to the Education and Training of All Nurses</u>
Occupational health nursing educators—in collaboration with staff from other disciplines (e.g., industrial hygiene, occupational medicine, engineering), NIOSH, AAOHN, and other expert

sources—should ensure that essential respiratory protection content is included in graduate occupational health nursing programs and integrated into continuing education courses for OHNs. The essential respiratory protection content should

- reiterate the value of respiratory protection in reducing illness and injury;
- reinforce respiratory protection throughout the graduate occupational health curriculum and clinical practice;
- include content on hazard assessment; respirator selection, use, care, and maintenance; medical evaluation and monitoring; respirator fit testing; employee training; and program evaluation;
- require, at a minimum, familiarity with relevant federal (e.g., 29 CFR 1910.134), state (e.g., Cal OSHA 5144), and national consensus (e.g., ANSI/AIHA Z88.10) regulations and standards;
- use hands-on education and training experiences to provide an understanding of the types of respirators and their uses;
- require students to demonstrate knowledge and skills in developing a respiratory protection program that includes training and evaluation components;
- emphasize the leadership role of OHNs in establishing a culture of safety, influencing behavior change and decisions related to respiratory and overall health, and promoting proper use of respirators in the workplace;
- examine research and best practices relevant to respiratory protection, behavioral change and leadership, and establishing a culture of safety in the workplace;
- consider including spirometry certification as a requirement for graduation; and
- specify elements that could be adapted and applied to continuing education programs and to the education and training of all nurses.

Teaching Methods and Resources for Respiratory Protection Education and Training

To successfully cover the essential content for a respiratory protection curriculum, occupational health nursing programs can use a range of approaches and resources to improve access to their courses and enhance the students' learning experience. Some occupational health nursing programs are already using innovative online and simulation educational methods to teach respiratory protection (e.g., Brown, 2011; Rupe, 2011).

Online courses offer an accessible format for students who do not have a school nearby. Of the OHNs surveyed by Mackey and colleagues (2003), over 56 percent reported that distance from a campus was a barrier to their obtaining a graduate degree. Online courses, including virtual lectures and training, webinars, Internet videoconferencing, and computer-managed instruction, are increasingly available and are being integrated into traditionally campus-based programs. Advantages and disadvantages of the distance learning approach were noted in the IOM's report *Safe Work in the 21st Century* (2000). Advantages include the program's ability to be flexible, to be reproduced, and to draw on experts at multiple institutions. Disadvantages include limited interaction with faculty and other students and the need to arrange for in-person activities, such as hands-on exercises and preceptorships. Students enrolled in an online course at schools such as the University of Iowa, where 50 percent of occupational health nursing students are out of state, are required to attend some courses in person (Rupe, 2011). This approach allows the students to take advantage of the flexibility of an online course yet also learn from applied activities.

Participants at the IOM workshop also described the value of using nontraditional teaching methods—such as simulation techniques, case studies, field observation and practice, and team projects—in addition to conventional classroom lectures. By using a range of teaching methods, education and training programs can more effectively convey and reinforce knowledge and skills in ways that target different learning styles and needs in order to better teach the essential content for respiratory protection. Presenters at the workshop emphasized the importance of hands-on educational approaches for effectively teaching OHNs how to use a respirator and how to instruct others in respirator use and maintenance. Hands-on learning experiences with fit testing and using a variety of respirators help OHNs understand the practical challenges presented by this equipment and the pros and cons of different models. Using a respirator while attempting to go about normal work-related tasks under normal working conditions is valuable in understanding worker concerns and experiences (Bayer, 2011).

Furthermore, using innovative teaching methods may help to emphasize the value of respirators and respiratory protection more broadly. Carrico and colleagues (2007) found that emergency department nurses who received a training program that involved a biosimulation of respiratory disease transmission, combined with standard classroom training, had a 74 percent rate of compliance with PPE use, compared to a 53 percent rate for a control group that received standard classroom training alone. Although the goal of this study was to evaluate PPE compliance when visual demonstration is used as a teaching approach, the study also noted that biosimulators are being used "to assist and improve the learning of residents, medical students, nursing students, and employed HCWs [health care workers]" and that the "visual demonstration [used in the study was] built on the principles of adult learning" (Carrico et al., 2007, p. 18). Comparable simulations could be useful in improving OHNs' abilities to teach workers about respiratory protection. Further efforts are needed to implement and evaluate a range of teaching methods to better meet the needs of occupational health nursing students.

Recommendation 5: <u>Develop, Expand, and Evaluate Innovative Teaching Methods and Resources to Establish Best Practices</u> Occupational health nursing education programs and respiratory protection programs should do the following:

- **Integrate essential content on respiratory protection into their core curricula and continuing education programs through a variety of innovative approaches, taking into consideration the needs of the students. These methods could include**

  o **online courses (including webinars),**
  o **simulation techniques,**
  o **case studies,**
  o **education and training modules,**
  o **field observation and practice, and**
  o **conferences and workshops.**

- **Draw on resources available from NIOSH, OSHA, state and local governments, the NIOSH ERCs and other**

educational institutions, professional organizations and unions, advocacy organizations, international health and safety organizations (e.g., the Network of World Health Organization Collaborating Centres in Occupational Health and the International Labour Organization), contractors, other professional communities and institutions, and the private sector.

- **Collaborate with NPPTL to evaluate innovative teaching methods used for respiratory protection education and training, including continuing education, in order to establish best practices in the field.**

Online Resources and Modules

Online resources, available through NIOSH and OSHA (http://www. cdc.gov/niosh and http://www.osha.gov), provide a wealth of information for occupational health and safety professionals. These websites include information on workplace safety and occupational hazards, such as flu preparedness and respirable dust exposure. Among other laws and regulations, OSHA's website includes the full text of 29 CFR 1910.134. Both NIOSH's and OSHA's websites have a number of respirator-specific resources that include information about respirators, respiratory protection, instructions and checklists for compliance with OSHA regulations, and opportunities for training and continuing education.

The NIOSH website could play a more active role in educating and training OHNs in respiratory protection. For example, it could highlight continuing education opportunities in respiratory protection and could offer additional resources for education and training purposes, such as case studies that illustrate the importance of respiratory protection and the value of respirators. NIOSH could also draw on the experiences of ERCs and develop content modules based on their best practices. If these modules were available and accessible on the NIOSH website, occupational health nursing programs could use them as a template or foundation for their curricula, and undergraduate nursing programs could use them to augment their curricula with respiratory protection content. Additionally, these content modules would allow OHNs who work in diverse settings to find information and tailor their learning experience to their specific work functions. By centralizing the resources in an easy-to-find place and supplementing with case studies and modules, NIOSH's website would be a valuable resource for educating and training OHNs.

Recommendation 6: <u>Expand Online Resources, Particularly Case Studies</u>
NPPTL should develop and maintain online resources for respiratory protection that are relevant to educating and training OHNs, specifically by

- **developing template modules that could be used in the core curriculum for occupational health nursing programs and that would draw on best practices of the NIOSH ERCs (sections of these modules could also be used for nursing students at all levels);**
- **compiling case studies (e.g., health hazard evaluations) that illustrate the value of respirators in protecting the health of workers across a range of work environments; and**
- **providing easily accessible links to existing resources, including the OSHA checklists.**

INCENTIVES FOR RESPIRATORY PROTECTION EDUCATION AND TRAINING

Making changes to graduate-level curricula or continuing education programs can be a significant endeavor requiring careful consideration of the justifications for change and the potential impact on cost, time, and educational resources. Improving respiratory protection curricula to ensure that OHNs are knowledgeable and feel confident in their skills will require a multifaceted approach and collaboration among a variety of professional organizations, educators, employers, government agencies, and OHNs. Incentives to improve and promote respiratory protection education and training can help drive change at the individual, educational, and employer levels. For example, the value and importance of respiratory protection could be further promoted through conferences, materials, and webinars that are hosted by professional associations, NIOSH, OSHA, and other organizations. Specific steps toward developing incentives and increasing awareness could include

- educational workshops at occupational health and safety professional meetings and conferences, such as those hosted by national organizations (e.g., AAOHN, AIHA, American College of Occupational and Environmental Medicine, American Public Health Association) and state and local affiliate groups, among others;
- workplace reviews of case studies and lessons learned from experiences on the value of respiratory protection;
- interdisciplinary activities within and outside NIOSH ERCs that emphasize respiratory protection; and
- focused efforts to include respiratory protection in research, educational, and clinical activities as part of master's and doctoral programs for nurses.

Incentives for improving respiratory protection knowledge and skills would by created if professional (e.g., AAOHN, ABOHN) and organizational (e.g., Joint Commission) accreditation and credentialing programs increased emphasis on respiratory protection. AAOHN develops and quadrennially updates a set of occupational health nursing competencies, which are used as the basis for curriculum development and the development of the ABOHN certification examination (AAOHN, 2007). The AAOHN competencies are divided into nine broad categories: (1) clinical practice; (2) case management; (3) workforce, workplace, and the environment; (4) regulatory or legislative; (5) management, business, and leadership; (6) health promotion and disease prevention; (7) health and safety education and training; (8) research; and (9) professionalism (AAOHN, 2007). The competencies highlight safety but do not focus on respiratory protection or other types of PPE; they are written broadly to cover the range of occupational health nursing practices that are integral to the work of OHNs. The committee suggests that AAOHN consider emphasizing knowledge of PPE and its appropriate use as a core competency. ABOHN, which offers certification exams, could then place a greater emphasis on questions relevant to PPE, including respiratory protection and respirators.

AAOHN (2006b) has also developed the *Core Curriculum for Occupational and Environmental Health Nursing* to guide occupation health nursing programs in developing their curricula. The AAOHN core curriculum includes information on respiratory protection. However, its focus is on the relevant federal regulations (AAOHN, 2006b). Further emphasis in the core curriculum on the value of respiratory protection for nurses themselves as well as workers, on the consequences of not using appropriate respiratory protection, and on instilling a culture of safety (including curricular components on behavioral and organizational change and leadership) would enhance this resource. Revisions to the AAOHN core curriculum and competencies with specificity regarding respiratory protection could potentially influence curricular changes. NPPTL could facilitate action toward these goals by exploring the development of core competencies that focus specifically on respiratory protection.

Recommendation 7: <u>Explore the Development of a Set of Core Competencies in Respiratory Protection</u>
NPPTL, in collaboration with relevant professional organizations, should explore the development of a set of interdisciplinary core competencies in respiratory protection that could be used to guide the education and training of OHNs and other occupational health and safety professionals.

A further emphasis on the proper use of PPE, including respirators, in organizational accreditation would signal the importance of knowledge and skills in respiratory protection. In addition to OSHA regulations requiring respiratory protection programs for workplaces with potential respiratory hazards, other worksite inspection and accreditation criteria influence the culture of workplace safety and the degree of emphasis placed on respiratory protection. For hospitals and other health care settings, Joint Commission standards are a key driver of quality improvement. Requirements for an infection control program are currently a part of the Joint Commission's criteria. Focused attention on PPE and respiratory protection by the Joint Commission could promote consistent respiratory protection practices in health care facilities and add an emphasis on and incentive for improving knowledge and skills in respiratory protection.

A 2008 IOM report stated that "[a] Joint Commission initiative focused on PPE compliance would be an immediate action that could have significant ramifications in improving awareness and appropriate use of PPE" (IOM, 2008, pp. 155-156). Further, the committee endorses the recommendation of the 2008 report: "Appropriate PPE use and healthcare worker safety should be a priority for healthcare organizations and healthcare workers, and in accreditation, regulatory policy, and training. Healthcare accrediting and credentialing organizations should ensure that

PPE training is part of the accreditation and testing curricula of health professional schools of nursing, medicine, and allied health and that PPE concepts and practice are included on certification examinations and as continuing education training requirements" (IOM, 2008, p. 140).

CONCLUSIONS

As key members of an occupational and environmental health and safety effort, OHNs contribute to the nation's health and productivity by helping to protect workers' health. Their knowledge, skill, and experience in respiratory protection are vital to protecting and promoting the nation's health and security during emergency and disaster situations, such as pandemic flu, severe acute respiratory syndrome, and terrorist events. OHNs partner with occupational medicine physicians, industrial hygienists, safety engineers, infection preventionists, and other dedicated health and safety professionals to promote and advance respiratory protection. These essential roles and responsibilities require OHNs who are well informed, engaged, and proficient in respiratory protection principles, practice, and motivation.

REFERENCES

AAOHN (American Association of Occupational Health Nurses). 2006a. *2006 compensation and benefits study: A statistical survey of job profiles, salaries and benefits.* Atlanta, GA: AAOHN.

———. 2006b. *Core curriculum for occupational and environmental health nursing.* Third ed. St. Louis, MO: Saunders Elsevier.

———. 2007. Competencies in occupational and environmental health nursing. *Journal of the American Association of Occupational Health Nurses* 55(11):442-447.

———. 2011. *The occupational and environmental health nursing profession.* https://www.aaohn.org/fact-sheets/the-occupational-and-environmental-health-nursing-profession.html (accessed April 11, 2011).

ABOHN (American Board for Occupational Health Nurses). 2004. *Occupational health nursing safety management examination handbook.* http://www.goamp.com/Publications/candidateHandbooks/abohn-cohn-s-handbook.pdf (accessed July 5, 2011).

———. 2008a. *COHN-S examination candidate handbook.* http://www.goamp.com/Publications/candidateHandbooks/abohn-cohn-s-handbook.pdf (accessed July 5, 2011).

————. 2008b. *COHN examination candidate handbook.* http://www.goamp. com/Publications/candidateHandbooks/abohn-cohn-handbook.pdf (accessed July 5, 2011).

————. 2009. *Case management examination candidate handbook.* http://www. goamp.com/Publications/candidateHandbooks/abohn-cm-handbook.pdf (accessed July 5, 2011).

ANA (American Nurses Association). 2010. *Code of ethics for nurses with interpretive statements.* http://www.nursingworld.org/MainMenuCategories/ EthicsStandards/CodeofEthicsforNurses/Code-of-Ethics.aspx (accessed May 6, 2011).

Banga, A., M. J. Reilly, and K. D. Rosenman. 2011. A study of characteristics of Michigan workers with work-related asthma exposed to welding. *Journal of Occupational and Environmental Medicine* 53(4):415-419.

Bayer, F. 2011. *Respiratory protection curriculum for occupational health nursing programs: PowerPoint presented at the IOM Workshop on Respiratory Protection Curriculum for Occupational Health Nursing Programs in Pittsburgh, PA.* http://iom.edu/~/media/Files/Activity%20Files/Education/ RespiratoryProtectionNurses/Panel%203-4%20Bayer.pdf (accessed May 6, 2011).

Brown, K. 2011. *Respiratory protection curriculum for OHN students at the University of Alabama at Birmingham: PowerPoint presented at the IOM Workshop on Respiratory Protection Curriculum for Occupational Health Nursing Programs in Pittsburgh, PA.* http://iom.exu/~/media/Files/Activity %20Files/Education/RespiratoryProtectionNurses/Panel%201-4%20Brown. pdf (accessed July 6, 2011).

Buckheit, K. 2011. *Respiratory protection for nurses—University of North Carolina at Chapel Hill: PowerPoint presented at the IOM Workshop on Respiratory Protection Curriculum for Occupational Health Nursing Programs in Pittsburgh, PA.* http://iom.edu/~/media/Files/Activity%20Files/Education/ RespiratoryProtectionNurses/Panel%202-1%20Buckheit.pdf (accessed May 5, 2011).

Burns, C. 2011. *Respiratory protection curriculum—University of South Florida: PowerPoint presented at the IOM Workshop on Respiratory Protection Curriculum for Occupational Health Nursing Programs in Pittsburgh, PA.* http://iom.edu/~/media/Files/Activity%20Files/Education/RespiratoryProtection Nurses/Panel%201-1%20Burns.pdf (accessed May 5, 2011).

Carpenter, H. 2011. *Respiratory protection—continuing education for registered nurses: PowerPoint presented at the IOM Workshop on Respiratory Protection Curriculum for Occupational Health Nursing Programs in Pittsburgh, PA.* http://iom.edu/~/media/Files/Activity%20Files/Education/RespiratoryProtection Nurses/Panel%202-3%20Carpenter.pdf (accessed May 6, 2011).

Carrico, R. M., M. B. Coty, L. K. Goss, and A. S. Lajoie. 2007. Changing health care worker behavior in relation to respiratory disease transmission with a novel training approach that uses biosimulation. *American Journal of Infection Control* 35(1):14-19.

CDC (Centers for Disease Control and Prevention). 2010. Occupational transmission of *Neisseria meningitidis*—California, 2009. *Morbidity and Mortality Weekly Report* 59(45):1480-1483.

Davis, S. 2011. *Current respiratory curricula at the University of Cincinnati College of Nursing: PowerPoint presented at the IOM Workshop on Respiratory Protection Curriculum for Occupational Health Nursing Programs in Pittsburgh, PA.* http://iom.edu/~/media/Files/Activity%20Files/Education/RespiratoryProtectionNurses/Panel%201-2%20Davis.pdf (accessed May 5, 2011).

Donham, K. J., J. L. Lange, A. Kline, R. H. Rautiainen, and L. Grafft. 2011. Prevention of occupational respiratory symptoms among certified safe farm intervention participants. *Journal of Agromedicine* 16(1):40-51.

Hofmann, D. A., R. Jacobs, and F. Landy. 1995. High reliability process industries: Individual, micro, and macro organizational influences on safety performance. *Journal of Safety Research* 26(3):131-149.

HRSA (Health Resources and Services Administration). 2006. *The registered nurse population: Findings from the March 2004 National Sample Survey of Registered Nurses.* http://bhpr.hrsa.gov/healthworkforce/rnsurveys/rnsurvey2004.pdf (accessed July 5, 2011).

———. 2010. *The registered nurse population: Findings from the 2008 National Sample Survey of Registered Nurses.* http://bhpr.hrsa.gov/healthworkforce/rnsurveys/rnsurveyfinal.pdf (accessed July 5, 2011).

IOM (Institute of Medicine). 2000. *Safe work in the 21st century: Education and training needs for the next decade's occupational safety and health personnel.* Washington, DC: National Academy Press.

———. 2003. *Health professions education: A bridge to quality.* Washington, DC: The National Academies Press.

———. 2008. *Preparing for an influenza pandemic: Personal protective equipment for healthcare workers.* Washington, DC: The National Academies Press.

———. 2011. *The future of nursing: Leading change, advancing health.* Washington, DC: The National Academies Press.

Mackey, T. A., F. L. Cole, and S. Parnell. 2003. Occupational health nurses' educational needs: What do they want? *American Association of Occupational Health Nurses Journal* 51(12):514-520.

Maples, E. 2011. *Deep South Center for Occupational Health and Safety: PowerPoint presented at the IOM Workshop on Respiratory Protection Curriculum for Occupational Health Nursing Programs in Pittsburgh, PA.* http://iom.edu/~/media/Files/Activity%20Files/Education/RespiratoryProtectionNurses/Panel%202-2%20Maples.pdf (accessed May 5, 2011).

McCullagh, M. 2011. *Respiratory protection curriculum—University of Michigan Occupational Health Nursing Program: PowerPoint presented at the*

IOM Workshop on Respiratory Protection Curriculum for Occupational Health Nursing Programs in Pittsburgh, PA. http://iom.edu/~/media/Files/Activity%20Files/Education/RespiratoryProtectionNurses/Panel%201-3%20 McCullagh.pdf (accessed May 5, 2011).

NIOSH (National Institute for Occupational Safety and Health). 2009. *About NPPTL*. http://www.cdc.gov/niosh/npptl/about.html (accessed May 5, 2011).

———. 2011a. *Health hazard evaluations: Frequently asked questions*. http://www.cdc.gov/niosh/hhe/faq.html (accessed May 5, 2011).

———. 2011b. *List of NIOSH education and research centers (ERCs)*. http://www.cdc.gov/niosh/oep/centers.html (accessed April 11, 2011).

———. 2011c. *NIOSH education and research centers (ERCs)*. http://www.cdc.gov/niosh/oep/cedirlst.html (accessed April 11, 2011).

North Carolina Division of Public Health. 2011. Respiratory protection curriculum content: Data gathering, submitted to the IOM Committee, March 16.

Oestenstad, R. K. 2010. *The Deep South Center for Occupational Health and Safety, Summary Annual Report July 1, 2009-June 30, 2010: NIOSH training grant T42OH008436*. Birmingham, AL: Deep South Center for Occupational Health and Safety.

OSHA (Occupational Safety and Health Administration). 2011. *Respiratory protection*. http://www.osha.gov/SLTC/respiratoryprotection/index.html (accessed April 7, 2011).

Rice, C., and T. Reponen. 2010. *University of Cincinnati Education and Research Center for Occupational Safety and Health, Summary Annual Report: July 1, 2009-June 30, 2010: NIOSH training grant T42OH008436*. Cincinnati, OH: University of Cincinnati Education and Research Center for Occupational Safety and Health.

Robbins, W. 2011. *Southern California Education and Research Center—Occupational and Environmental Health Nursing (OEHN) Program at the University of California, Los Angeles: PowerPoint presented at the IOM Workshop on Respiratory Protection Curriculum for Occupational Health Nursing Programs in Pittsburgh, PA*. http://iom.edu/~/media/Files/Activity %20Files/Education/RespiratoryProtectionNurses/Panel%201-5%20Robbins.pdf (accessed May 5, 2011).

Rupe, K. 2011. *Respiratory protection curriculum—University of Iowa College of Nursing: PowerPoint presented at the IOM Workshop on Respiratory Protection Curriculum for Occupational Health Nursing Programs in Pittsburgh, PA*. http://iom.edu/~/media/Files/Activity%20Files/Education/ Respiratory ProtectionNurses/Panel%201-6%20Rupe%20v2.pdf (accessed May 5, 2011).

Ryan, M. G. 2001. Developing a respiratory protection program. Understanding the written elements. *American Association of Occupational Health Nurses Journal* 49(6):293-307; quiz 308-309.

Strasser, P. B., H. K. Maher, G. Knuth, and L. J. Fabrey. 2006. Occupational health nursing 2004 practice analysis report. *American Association of Occupational Health Nurses Journal* 54(1):14-23.

Thompson, M. C. 2010. Review of occupational health nurse data from recent National Sample Surveys of Registered Nurses—part I. *American Association of Occupational Health Nurses Journal* 58(1):27-39.

Townsend, M. 2011a. *NIOSH-approved spirometry training.* http://www.mctownsend.com (accessed July 6, 2011).

———. 2011b. *Respiratory protection training for OHNs—developing a one-day fit-testing workshop: PowerPoint presented at the IOM Workshop on Respiratory Protection Curriculum for Occupational Health Nursing Programs in Pittsburgh, PA.* http://iom.edu/~/media/Files/Activity%20Files/Education/RespiratoryProtectionNurses/Panel%203-1%20Townsend.pdf (accessed May 6, 2011).

UCLA (University of California, Los Angeles) School of Public Health. 2011. Respiratory protection curriculum content: Data gathering from NIOSH ERC Nursing Programs, submitted to the IOM Committee, March 16.

UCSF (University of California, San Francisco). 2011. Respiratory protection curriculum content: Data gathering from NIOSH ERC Nursing Programs, submitted to the IOM Committee, March 16.

University of Alabama at Birmingham School of Nursing. 2011. Respiratory protection curriculum content: Data gathering from NIOSH ERC Nursing Programs, submitted to the IOM Committee, March 16.

University of Iowa College of Public Health. 2011. Respiratory protection curriculum content: Data gathering from NIOSH ERC Nursing Programs, submitted to the IOM Committee, March 16.

University of Michigan School of Nursing. 2011. Respiratory protection curriculum content: Data gathering from NIOSH ERC Nursing Programs, submitted to the IOM Committee, March 16.

University of South Florida College of Public Health. 2011. Respiratory protection curriculum content: Data gathering from NIOSH ERC Nursing Programs, submitted to the IOM Committee, March 16.

A

Workshop Agenda

March 30, 2011
Hyatt Regency Pittsburgh International Airport
Pittsburgh, Pennsylvania

*Workshop on Respiratory Protection Curriculum for
Occupational Health Nursing Programs*

OPEN SESSION

8:00 a.m. **Coffee Available**

8:30 **Welcome and Introductions**
      Linda Hawes Clever and Bonnie Rogers, Co-Chairs,
      IOM Committee on the Respiratory Protection
      Curriculum for Occupational Health Nursing Programs

8:45 **Perspective from the National Personal Protective
      Technology Laboratory (NPPTL)**
      Maryann D'Alessandro, Associate Director for Science,
      NPPTL

9:00   **Panel 1: Current Respiratory Protection Curricula**

Facilitator: *Bonnie Rogers*

9:00-9:05	Panel Introductions
9:05-9:15	*Candace Burns*, University of South Florida
9:15-9:25	*Sue Davis*, University of Cincinnati
9:25-9:35	*Marjorie McCullagh*, University of Michigan
9:35-9:45	*Kathleen Brown*, University of Alabama at Birmingham
9:45-9:55	*Wendie Robbins*, University of California, Los Angeles
9:55-10:05	*Kerri Rupe*, University of Iowa
10:05-10:45	Discussion with the committee

Questions:

- *What is the current respiratory protection curriculum at your institution? What course(s) incorporates this training? Who teaches this segment? How much time is devoted to respiratory protection?*
- *In what way could the respiratory protection curriculum be enhanced?*
- *Are there any barriers or challenges that need to be overcome to improve the training to produce professionals who are fully aware and informed about respiratory protection technologies and who can teach and model the use of respiratory protection? How might barriers be surmounted?*

10:45   **Break**

11:00   **Panel 2: Continuing Education and Occupational Health Nursing Boards and Organizations**

Facilitator: *Barbara DeBaun*

11:00-11:05	Panel Introductions
11:05-11:15	*Kathleen Buckheit*, University of North Carolina at Chapel Hill

11:15-11:25	*Elizabeth Maples,* University of Alabama at Birmingham
11:25-11:35	*Holly Carpenter,* American Nurses Association
11:35-11:45	*Kathleen Buckheit,* American Association of Occupational Health Nurses
11:45-11:55	*Pam Hart,* American Board of Occupational Health Nurses
11:55-12:30	Discussion with the committee

Questions:

- *What efforts are being made in nursing continuing education programs regarding respiratory protection training? In what way could the respiratory protection content be enhanced?*
- *Are there any barriers or challenges that need to be overcome to improve the continuing education training? How might barriers be surmounted?*
- *What efforts are or could be conducted by national associations and boards to increase awareness and training on respiratory protection?*
- *Are there instructor certification or other mechanisms that should be considered in ensuring quality instruction?*

12:30 p.m. Lunch

1:15   Panel 3: Opportunities for Improving Respiratory Protection Training

Facilitator: *Patty Quinlan*

1:15-1:20	Panel Introductions
1:20-1:30	*Mary Townsend,* M. C. Townsend Associates
1:30-1:40	*Mark Tanis,* University of Pittsburgh Medical Center
1:40-1:50	*Tina Williams,* U.S. Army National Guard
1:50-2:00	*Felicia Bayer,* Alcoa
2:00-2:10	*Theresa Vaneman,* BASF
2:10-2:45	Discussion with the committee

Questions:
- *What respiratory protection programs are in place at your facility? Who is in charge of the programs? Where is the respiratory protection program in your organizational structure? What are the barriers to enhancing the respiratory protection program at your institution and how could any barriers be surmounted?*
- *How could nursing graduate programs and continuing education programs be enhanced to produce professionals who are fully aware and informed about respiratory protection technologies and who can teach and model the use of respiratory protection?*

2:45   Discussion—Ideas on Improving Respiratory Protection Curricula

Facilitator: *Linda Hawes Clever*

- Comments from audience members
- Discussion with panelists, audience, committee members
- Summary—*Linda Hawes Clever and Bonnie Rogers*

3:30   Adjourn Workshop

B

Workshop Participants

Members of the Institute of Medicine (IOM) Committee on the Respiratory Protection Curriculum for Occupational Health Nursing Programs

Linda Hawes Clever, *Co-Chair*
California Pacific Medical
   Center

M. E. Bonnie Rogers, *Co-Chair*
University of North Carolina at
   Chapel Hill

Edie Alfano-Sobsey
Region 4 Wake County Human
   Services

Barbara DeBaun
Cynosure Healthcare
   Consultants

Oisaeng Hong
University of California,
   San Francisco

Leslie M. Israel
University of California, Irvine

James S. Johnson
JSJ and Associates

Hernando R. Perez
Drexel University

Patricia Quinlan
University of California,
   San Francisco

IOM Project Staff

Catharyn T. Liverman

Andrea M. Schultz

Larisa M. Andersen

Workshop Presenters

Felicia Bayer
Alcoa, Inc.

Kathleen Brown
University of Alabama at
   Birmingham

Kathleen Buckheit
University of North Carolina at
   Chapel Hill

Candace Burns
University of South Florida

Holly Carpenter
American Nurses Association

L. Sue Davis
University of Cincinnati

Pam Hart
Doherty Employment Group

Elizabeth Maples
University of Alabama
   at Birmingham

Marjorie McCullagh
University of Michigan

Wendie Robbins
University of California, Los
   Angeles

Kerri Rupe
University of Iowa

Mark Tanis
University of Pittsburgh
   Medical Center

Mary C. Townsend
M. C. Townsend Associates,
   LLC

Theresa Vaneman
BASF

Tina Williams
U.S. Army National Guard

Members of the IOM Standing Committee on Personal Protective Equipment for Workplace Safety and Health

Charles Austin
Sheet Metal Occupational
   Health Institute Trust

Roger Barker
North Carolina State University

Robert Bass
Maryland Institute for
   Emergency Medical Services

David M. DeJoy
University of Georgia

Sundaresan Jayaraman
Georgia Institute of Technology

Knut Ringen
Independent Consultant

Anugrah Shaw
University of Maryland
at Eastern Shore

Daniel Shipp
International Safety Equipment
Association

James Tacci
Xerox Corporation

Participants

Jeffrey Birkner
Moldex-Metric, Inc.

Michele Bruer
Vanderbilt University

Charlotte Carneiro
Occupational Safety and Health
Administration, Office of
Occupational Health Nursing

Lisa Casanova
Georgia State University

Kyungim Jacob Cho
University of Cincinnati

Craig Colton
3M

Lorraine Conroy
University of Illinois at Chicago

Scott Cormier
Hospital Corporation of
America

Kate Durand
California Department of Public
Health

Ben Favret III
Vestagen Technical Textiles

Marta Figueroa
University of Medicine and
Dentistry of New Jersey

John Fishbeck
The Joint Commission

John Franke
University of Illinois at Chicago

MaryAnn Gruden
Association of Occupational
Health Professionals

Lorraine Harkavy
U.S. Department of Health and
Human Services

Donald Largent
Air Techniques International

Nicole McCullough
3M

Mary Ogg
Association of periOperative
Registered Nurses

Charles John Palenik
Indiana University

Rodney Parker
Stryker

Sanchia Patrick
Kimberly-Clark

Robert Phalen
California State University, San
  Bernardino

Aaron Richardson
Battelle

Margaret Sietsema
University of Illinois at Chicago

Girish Srinivas
TDA Research, Inc.

Stephen Streed
Lee Memorial Health System

Mamoru Yanagiuchi
Shigematsu Works, Co., LTD

Sponsor Representatives

David Book
National Personal Protective
  Technology Laboratory
  (NPPTL)

Maryann D'Alessandro
NPPTL

F. Selcen Kilinc-Balci
NPPTL

Debra Novak
NPPTL

Jeff Peterson
NPPTL

Consultant

Neil Weisfeld
NEW Associates, LLC

C

Recent Institute of Medicine Reports Related to Personal Protective Equipment and Education Needs of the Workforce

Preventing Transmission of Pandemic Influenza and Other Viral Respiratory Diseases: Personal Protective Equipment for Healthcare Personnel—Update 2010 (IOM, 2011)

This report looked at the progress made since the Institute of Medicine report *Preparing for an Influenza Pandemic* (2008) and reiterated the importance of appropriate use of personal protective equipment (PPE) to ensure worker safety, including the use of respirators for health care personnel exposed to viral respiratory disease. The report's recommendations called for further research on influenza transmission and respirator effectiveness and design (including the development of powered air-purifying respirators for health care personnel) as well as additional research on strategies to promote a culture of safety and encourage the use of PPE.

Respiratory Protection for Healthcare Workers in the Workplace Against Novel H1N1 Influenza A: A Letter Report (IOM, 2009)

This letter report recommended that health care workers use fit tested N95 respirators when in close contact with individuals who have H1N1 influenza A or similar illnesses to prevent further transmission. This recommendation highlighted the responsibilities of both the employers and the workers in implementing effective and appropriate use of PPE in accordance with Occupational Safety and Health Administration regulations. A second recommendation called for additional research on influenza transmission, the current effectiveness of respirators, and improved respirator design.

Preparing for an Influenza Pandemic: Personal Protective Equipment for Healthcare Workers (IOM, 2008)

This report concluded that the health care community is not prepared to use PPE effectively in the event of an influenza pandemic. Its recommendations focused on three main areas for immediate action: (1) research on influenza transmission should be a priority; (2) a culture of worker safety, including correct use of PPE, should be promoted; and (3) PPE should be developed with the needs of the worker in mind. The committee noted that the ability of respirators to reduce the spread of the disease by protecting both the health care worker and the patient makes them an essential component of PPE policy in an influenza pandemic.

The Personal Protective Technology Program at NIOSH (IOM and NRC, 2008)

This report evaluated and affirmed the positive impact and value of the National Institute of Occupational Safety and Health's (NIOSH's) Personal Protective Technology Program in the improvement of occupational safety and health and the reduction of workplace injuries and illnesses. The committee assessed NIOSH's respirator certification program and recommended that this program continue to be enhanced. The committee also recommended that further research be done on the barriers (including human factors) to effective use of PPE as well as ways to overcome them.

Safe Work in the 21st Century: Education and Training Needs for the Next Decade's Occupational Safety and Health Personnel (IOM, 2000)

This report concluded that changes in the demographics of the American workforce and in the workplace can impede the implementation of health and safety programs in the workplace. These complicating factors will require the development and implementation of a more comprehensive curricula, multidisciplinary training opportunities, and new types of training programs. Its recommendations focus on improving overall educational and training opportunities for current and future occupational safety and health professionals, including occupational health nurses.

REFERENCES

IOM (Institute of Medicine). 2000. *Safe work in the 21st century: Education and training needs for the next decade's occupational safety and health personnel.* Washington, DC: National Academy Press.

———. 2008. *Preparing for an influenza pandemic: Personal protective equipment for healthcare workers.* Washington, DC: The National Academies Press.

———. 2009. *Respiratory protection for healthcare workers in the workplace against novel H1N1 Influenza A: A letter report.* Washington, DC: The National Academies Press.

———. 2011. *Preventing transmission of pandemic influenza and other viral respiratory diseases: Personal protective equipment for healthcare personnel—Update 2010.* Washington, DC: The National Academies Press.

IOM and NRC (National Research Council). 2008. *The personal protective technology program at NIOSH.* Washington, DC: The National Academies Press.

D

Committee Biographies

Linda Hawes Clever, M.D. (*Co-Chair*), is a specialist in internal medicine and occupational medicine. She attended undergraduate and medical school at Stanford University and did postdoctoral training at Stanford and the University of California, San Francisco (UCSF). She is a member of the Institute of Medicine (IOM) of the National Academy of Sciences; clinical professor of medicine at UCSF; associate dean for alumni affairs at the Stanford University School of Medicine; and founding chair and senior physician of the Division of Occupational Health at California Pacific Medical Center. She is also the founding president of RENEW, a not-for-profit aimed at helping devoted people maintain and regain enthusiasm, effectiveness, and purpose as they resolve the competing imperatives of work and life. Her husband is an internist as is their daughter, who is on the faculty at the Johns Hopkins School of Medicine. Dr. Clever served on the Stanford University Board of Trustees for 14 years and was editor of the *Western Journal of Medicine*; she also chaired the board of the public broadcasting station KQED. Dr. Clever speaks nationally and internationally and has many publications on topics including health promotion, occupational health, personal and institutional renewal, volunteerism, and leadership. Her book, *The Fatigue Prescription: Four Ways to Renewing Your Energy, Health, and Life*, was published in 2010.

M. E. Bonnie Rogers, Dr.P.H., COHN-S, LNCC, FAAN (*Co-Chair*), is an associate professor of nursing and public health and director of the North Carolina Occupational Safety and Health Education and Research Center and the Occupational Health Nursing Program at the University of North Carolina, School of Public Health, Chapel Hill. Dr. Rogers received her diploma in nursing from the Washington Hospital Center

School of Nursing, Washington, DC; her baccalaureate in nursing from George Mason University School of Nursing, Fairfax, Virginia; and her master of public health degree and doctorate in public health from the Johns Hopkins University School of Hygiene and Public Health. Dr. Rogers was a visiting scholar at the Hasting Center in New York and is an ethics consultant. Dr. Rogers serves as chairperson of the NIOSH National Occupational Research Agenda Liaison Committee. She has served on numerous IOM committees including the IOM Standing Committee on Personal Protective Equipment for Workplace Safety and Health. Dr. Rogers is past president of the American Association of Occupational Health Nurses and the Association of Occupational and Environmental Clinics. She is currently Vice President of the International Commission on Occupational Health.

Edie Alfano-Sobsey, Ph.D., MT(ASCP), is currently a public health epidemiologist with Wake County Human Services in North Carolina. She recently served as an industrial hygienist, epidemiologist, and team leader of the NC Public Health Regional Surveillance Team 4. In this position, she was successful in creating and leading new initiatives in public health preparedness. These include developing the environmental sampling protocol for bioterrorism agents used by North Carolina public health and first responders, implementing and evaluating respiratory protection programs in health care agencies, developing and assisting with preparedness plans, creating training in epidemiology and outbreak investigation for local health departments, and coordinating exercises to test local and state preparedness plans. Dr. Alfano-Sobsey's other areas of expertise include infectious disease epidemiology, medical laboratory sciences (specializing in microbiology), and environmental health sciences, with peer-reviewed publications in these areas. She holds a doctor of philosophy in infectious disease epidemiology and a master of science in public health in environmental sciences, both from the University of North Carolina at Chapel Hill. She is also a certified medical technologist and clinical laboratory scientist.

Barbara DeBaun, R.N., M.S.N., CIC, has more than 30 years of experience in the field of infection prevention and control. She is currently an improvement advisor for Cynosure Healthcare Consultants. Prior to this role she supported BEACON, the Bay Area Patient Safety Collaborative where she provided vision and leadership in the development, implementation, and facilitation of performance improvement initiatives for the 38 participating medical centers in the San Francisco Bay Area. Previously, she was the director of patient safety and infection control at California Pacific Medical Center in San Francisco. Before that she directed the infection control programs at St. Mary's Medical Center in San Francisco and the VA Hospital in the Bronx, New York. She is a certified infection control practitioner and holds a bachelor's degree in nursing from Pace University in New York and a master of science degree in nursing from San Francisco State University. She is adjunct faculty at Dominican University California. She is an active member of the Association for Professionals in Infection Control and Epidemiology (APIC). Ms. DeBaun currently serves as the chair of the 2012 APIC Annual Conference Committee and is a member of the APIC Education Committee and the APIC Practice Guidance Council. She is the APIC liaison to the Centers for Disease Control and Prevention Hospital Infection Control Practices Advisory Committee. She has lectured nationally and internationally on a variety of patient safety and infection control topics and has published more than a dozen articles and several book chapters. In 2008, she was selected as *Infection Control Today's* Educator of the Year. Ms. DeBaun is a member of the IOM Standing Committee on Personal Protective Equipment for Workplace Safety and Health.

Oisaeng Hong, Ph.D., R.N., is professor in the Department of Community Health Systems and director of the Occupational and Environmental Health Nursing Program at the Northern California Center for Occupational and Environmental Health at UCSF. Her research focuses on the health and safety of workers with noise and chemical exposures and of underserved immigrant worker populations, with an emphasis on community and workplace-based participatory health interventions. Dr. Hong is a recognized expert in the prevention occupational hearing loss through a multidisciplinary hearing protection intervention research funded by NIOSH, the National Institutes of Health, and the Department of Homeland Security. Her intervention research adapts the concept of tailoring to provide information most relevant to individual workers and incorporates internet and mobile phone applications for wide dissemination in diverse worker populations. Dr. Hong's sustained research has contributed to knowledge development, practice, and policy making nationally and internationally through scholarly publications and presentations. Dr. Hong received her master of science in nursing from Yon Sei University (South Korea), her doctorate in nursing from the University of

Illinois at Chicago, and a postdoctoral fellowship in health promotion and risk reduction from the University of Michigan, Ann Arbor.

Leslie M. Israel, D.O., M.P.H., FACOEM, is an associate clinical professor in the Department of Medicine, Division of Occupational and Environmental Medicine at the University of California, Irvine. She received her internship and residency training at Yale University and is board-certified in occupational medicine. Dr. Israel serves as the associate director of the University of California, Irvine, Occupational Medicine Residency Program and medical director for the University of California, Center for Occupational and Environmental Health Occupational and Environmental Medicine Clinic. In addition, she is working on several clinical research projects: Firefighter Occupational Exposures in collaboration with the Biomonitoring California Program, a NIOSH-funded Firefighter Obesity Study (FORWARD), and a review of workers' compensation claims by firefighters for cardiac conditions. She serves as vice president of the Western Occupational Medicine Association (2011) and recently served as the chair for the National Occupational Medicine Residency Program Directors Group (May 1, 2010, to March 25, 2011). Dr. Israel is a member of the IOM Standing Committee on Personal Protective Equipment for Workplace Safety and Health.

James S. Johnson, Ph.D., CIH, QEP, has worked at the Lawrence Livermore National Laboratory (LLNL) since 1972. His position from November 2000 was section leader of the Chemical and Biological Safety Section of the Safety Programs Division. Throughout his career at LLNL, Dr. Johnson has been involved with respiratory protection and personal protective equipment as the respiratory program administrator, research scientist, and division and section manager. He is an American Industrial Hygiene Association (AIHA) fellow; a member of the National Fire Protection Association (NFPA) Technical Correlating Committee on Fire and Emergency Services Protective Clothing and Equipment; a member of the NFPA Respiratory Protection Equipment Committee; past chair of the International Society for Respiratory Protection, Americas Section; secretariat chair of the American National Standards Institute (ANSI) Z88 for Respiratory Protection; and a member and past chairman of the AIHA Respirator Committee. He is also a member of the AIHA Protective Clothing and Equipment Committee and the Emergency Preparedness and Response Task Force. Dr. Johnson retired from LLNL on July 1, 2006, and is now a part-time consultant. He has taught a one-semester industrial hygiene class at Chabot-Las Positas Community College since 1982 and a variety of respiratory protection training classes. Dr. Johnson is a member of the IOM Standing Committee on Personal Protective Equipment for Workplace Safety and Health.

Hernando R. Perez, Ph.D., M.P.H., CIH, is an assistant professor at the Drexel University School of Public Health. He received his master's of public health in environmental and occupational health from Emory University and his Ph.D. in industrial hygiene from Purdue University. Dr. Perez is certified in the comprehensive practice of industrial hygiene by the American Board of Industrial Hygiene and serves as director of the Drexel School of Public Health's industrial hygiene consulting service. He is also certified in safety by the Board of Certified Safety Professionals. His research interests include environmental and occupational bioaerosol assessment, children's environmental health, and housing and health. Dr. Perez served as consultant, facilitator, and report writer to the Mold Task Force of the Pennsylvania Department of Health. He has also collaborated with both the Philadelphia Department of Health and the Philadelphia Housing Authority on their Housing and Urban Development–funded Healthy Homes Demonstration Projects. Additionally, he has served as a grant reviewer for internal proposals at NIOSH, as well as a senior grant reviewer for Round 12 of the U.S. Department of Housing and Urban Development Lead Hazard Control Grant Program.

Patricia Quinlan, M.P.H., CIH, is an industrial hygienist–senior specialist in the School of Medicine at UCSF. She also holds an appointment as a clinical professor of nursing at UCSF School of Nursing. Her job duties include research, teaching, clinical support work, and community service. Over the past 24 years she has been involved with a series of research projects whose purpose is to better understand the impact of work and the environment on health—specifically how various agents may affect the health of workers and members of the public. These studies have included examining the neurotoxic effects of exposures to solvents and methanol and the pulmonary effects of exposure to agents such as aerosolized pentamidine and metal fumes. Other research has included evaluating workers' exposures for a retrospective colon cancer study, a study of gradients of health in hospital workers, and occupational exposure assessment for several population-based case-control studies of Parkinson's disease and childhood leukemia. Her current research includes studies regarding the effects of environmental exposures on subjects with asthma, chronic obstructive pulmonary disease, and hypersensitivity pneumonitis. Ms. Quinlan has served on several advisory committees for the California Occupational Safety and Health Administration, including the 5155 Air Contaminants Committee and the general advisory committee. She also is a member of the board of directors of Worksafe, a health and safety advocacy organization.